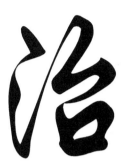

Visual Materia Medica of Chinese Herbs

Sacred Lotus Arts, Inc.

2nd Edition

Revision 1.0

Visual Materia Medica of Chinese Herbs

Table of Contents

bái zhǐ (Angelica Root)

白芷

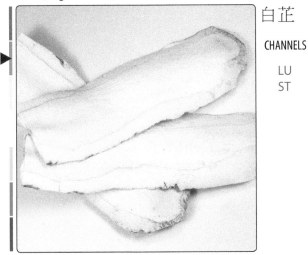

CHANNELS

LU
ST

Radix Angelicae Dahuricae
spicy, warm

fáng fēng (Ledebouriella Root)

防风

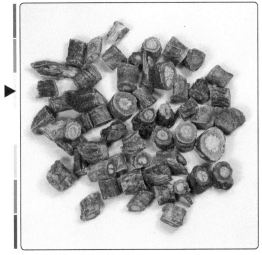

CHANNELS

BL
LIV
SP

Radix Ledebouriellae Divaricatae
spicy, sweet, slightly warm

gǎo běn (Straw Weed, Chinese Lovage Root)

藁本

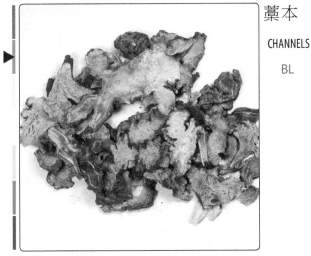

CHANNELS

BL

Radix et Rhizoma Ligustici Chinensis
spicy, warm

guì zhī (Cinnamon Twig, Cassia Twig)

桂枝

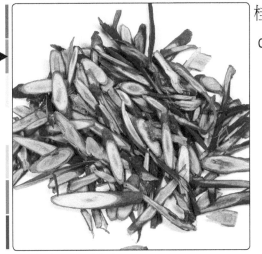

CHANNELS

HT
LU
BL

Ramulus Cinnamomi Cassiae
spicy, sweet, warm

jīng jiè (Schizonepeta Bud or Stem)

荆芥

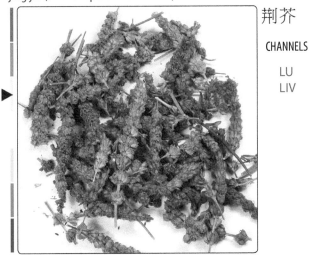

CHANNELS

LU
LIV

Herba Seu Flos Schizonepetae Tenuifoliae
spicy, aromatic, slightly warm

má huáng (Ephedra Stem)

麻黄

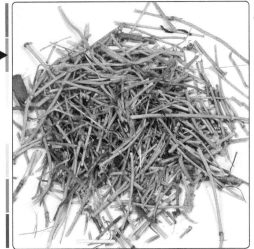

CHANNELS

LU
BL

Herba Ephedrae
spicy, slightly bitter, warm

Warm, Spicy Herbs that Release the Exterior

qiāng huó (Notopterygium Root)

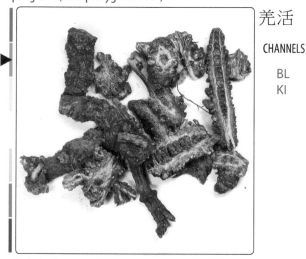

羌活

CHANNELS

BL
KI

Radix Et Rhizoma Notopterygii
spicy, bitter, aromatic, warm

shēng jiāng (Fresh Ginger Rhizome)

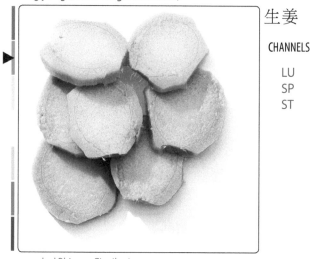

生姜

CHANNELS

LU
SP
ST

uncooked Rhizoma Zingiberis
spicy, warm

xì xīn (Chinese Wild Ginger, Asarum)

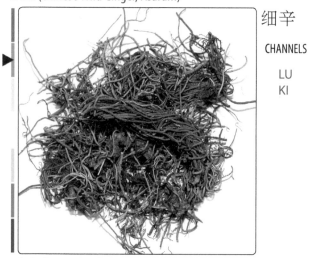

细辛

CHANNELS

LU
KI

Herba Asari Cum Radice
spicy, warm

xiāng rú (Aromatic Madder, Elsholtzia)

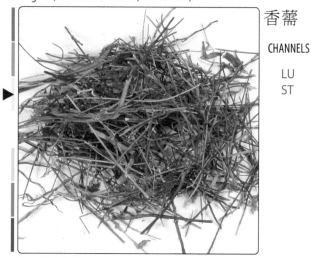

香薷

CHANNELS

LU
ST

Herba Elsholtziae
spicy, aromatic, slightly warm

xīn yí (Magnolia Flower)

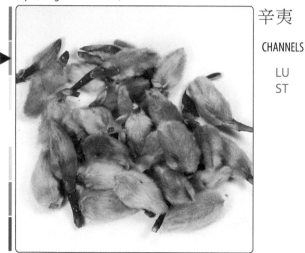

辛夷

CHANNELS

LU
ST

Flos Magnoliae Lilliflorae
spicy, warm

zǐ sū gěng (Perilla Stalk)

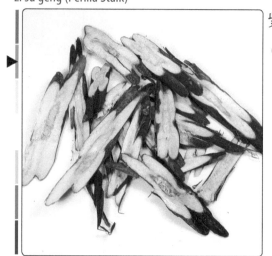

紫苏根

CHANNELS

LU
ST

Perillae Ramulus
spicy, warm

zǐ sū yè (Perilla Leaf)

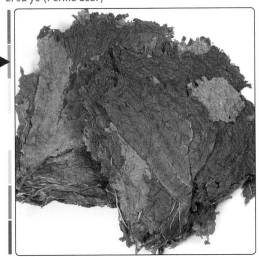

紫苏叶

CHANNELS

LU
SP

Perillae Folium
spicy, aromatic, warm

bò he (Field Mint, Mentha)

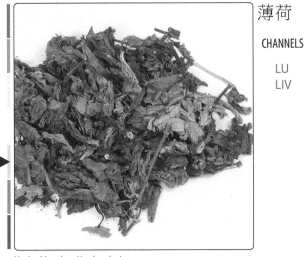

薄荷

CHANNELS

LU
LIV

Herba Menthae Haplocalycis
spicy, aromatic, cool

chái hú (Thorowax Root , Bupleurum)

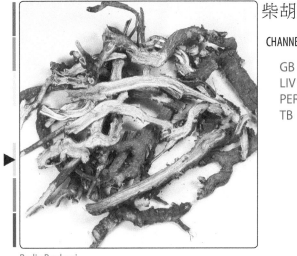

柴胡

CHANNELS

GB
LIV
PER
TB

Radix Bupleuri
bitter, spicy, cool

chán tuì (Circada Moulting)

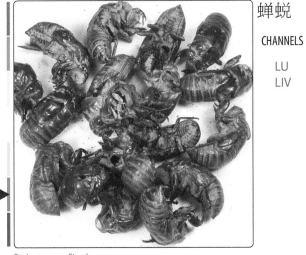

蝉蜕

CHANNELS

LU
LIV

Periostracum Cicadae
sweet, salty, slightly cold

dàn dòu chì (Prepared Soybean)

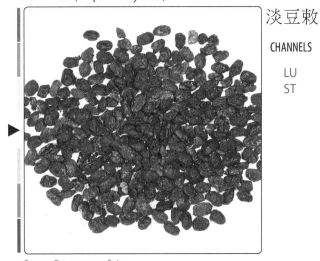

淡豆敊

CHANNELS

LU
ST

Semen Praeparatum Sojae
sweet, slightly bitter, neutral

fú píng (Duckweed or Spirodela)

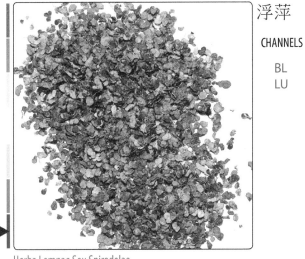

浮萍

CHANNELS

BL
LU

Herba Lemnae Seu Spirodelae
spicy, cold

gé gēn (Pueraria, Kudzu Root)

ye ge gen shown

葛根

CHANNELS

SP
ST

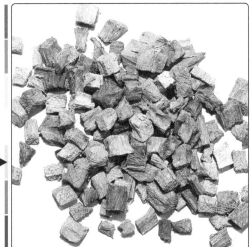

Radix Puerariae
sweet, spicy, cool

jú huā (Chrysanthemum Flower)

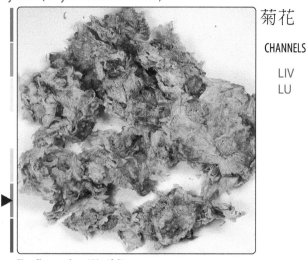

菊花

CHANNELS

LIV
LU

Flos Chrysanthemi Morifolii
sweet, bitter, slightly cold

màn jīng zǐ (Vitex Fruit)

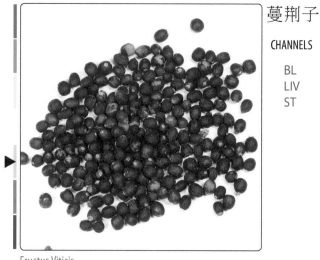

蔓荆子

CHANNELS

BL
LIV
ST

Fructus Viticis
bitter, spicy, cool

mù zéi (Shave Grass, Scouring Rush)

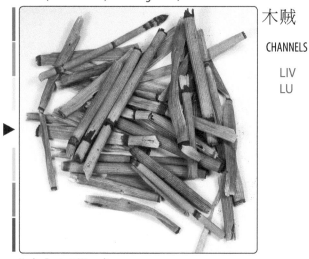

木贼

CHANNELS

LIV
LU

Herba Equiseti Hiemalis
sweet, bitter, neutral

niú bàng zǐ (Great Burdock Fruit)

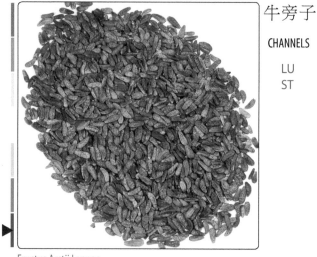

牛旁子

CHANNELS

LU
ST

Fructus Arctii Lappae
spicy, bitter, cold

sāng yè (White Mulberry Leaf)

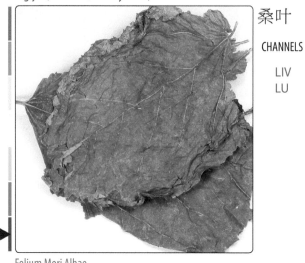

桑叶

CHANNELS

LIV
LU

Folium Mori Albae
sweet, bitter, cold

shēng má (Black Cohosh Rhizome, Bugbane Rhizome)

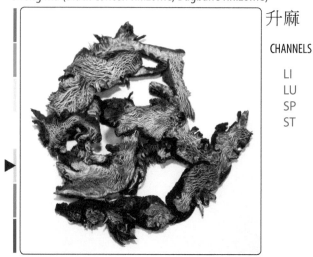

升麻

CHANNELS

LI
LU
SP
ST

Rhizoma Cimicifugae
sweet, spicy, cool

dàn zhú yè (Lophatherum Stem and Leaves)

淡竹叶

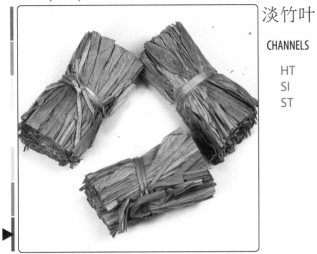

CHANNELS

HT
SI
ST

Herba Lophatheri Gracilis
sweet, bland, cold

gŭ jīng căo (Inflorscence or Pipewort Scapus)

谷精草

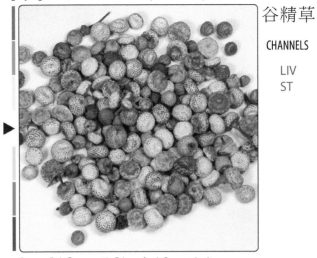

CHANNELS

LIV
ST

Scapus Et Inflorescentia Eriocaulonis Buergeriani
sweet, neutral

hán shuĭ shí (Calcitum)

寒水石

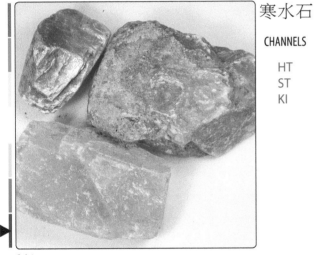

CHANNELS

HT
ST
KI

Calcitum
spicy, salty, cold

jué míng zĭ (Cassia or Foetid Cassia Seeds)

决明子

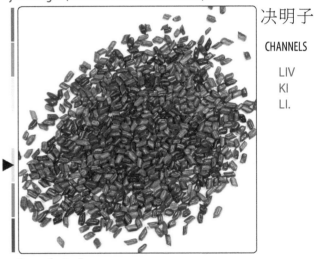

CHANNELS

LIV
KI
LI.

Semen Cassiae Torae
bitter, sweet, cool

lián zĭ xīn (Lotus Plumule)

连子心

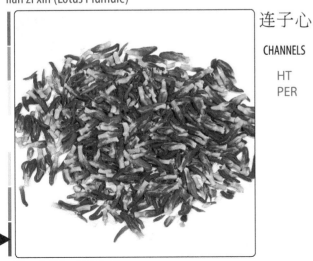

CHANNELS

HT
PER

Plumula Nelumbinis Nuciferae
bitter, cold

lú gēn (Reed Rhizome)

芦根

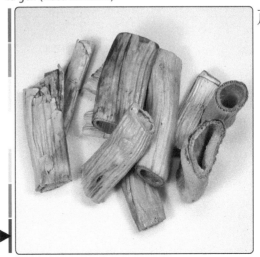

CHANNELS

LU
ST

Rhizoma Phragmitis Communis
sweet, cold

mì Méng huā (Buddleia Flower Bud)

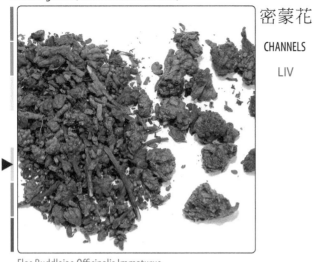

密蒙花

CHANNELS

LIV

Flos Buddleiae Officinalis Immaturus
sweet, cool

qīng xiāng zǐ (Celosia Seeds)

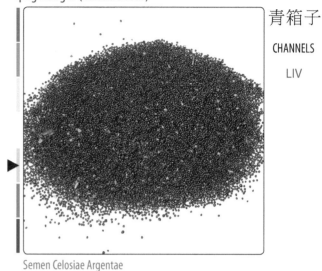

青箱子

CHANNELS

LIV

Semen Celosiae Argentae
sweet, cool

shí gāo (Gypsum)

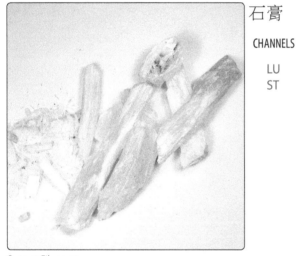

石膏

CHANNELS

LU
ST

Gypsum Fibrosum
sweet, spicy, very cold

xià kū cǎo (Prunella or Selfheal Spike)

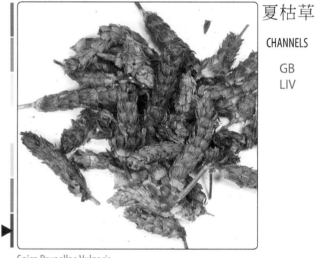

夏枯草

CHANNELS

GB
LIV

Spica Prunellae Vulgaris
bitter, spicy, cold

yè míng shā (Bat Feces)

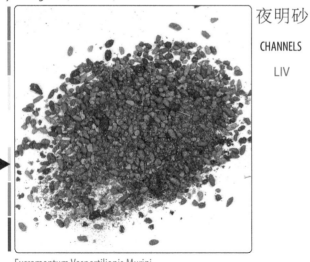

夜明砂

CHANNELS

LIV

Excrementum Vespertilionis Murini
spicy, cool

zhī mǔ (Anemarrhena Rhizome)

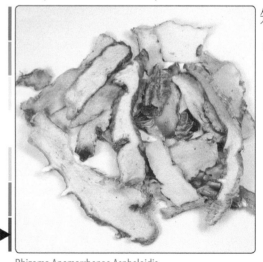

知母

CHANNELS

LU
ST
KI

Rhizoma Anemarrhenae Aspheloidis
bitter, cold

zhī zi (Gardenia, Cape Jasmine Fruit)

栀子

CHANNELS

HT
LIV
LU
ST
TB

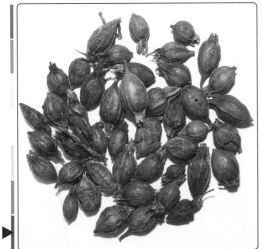

Fructus Gardeniae Jasminoidis
bitter, cold

bái wēi (Swallowwort Root)

白薇

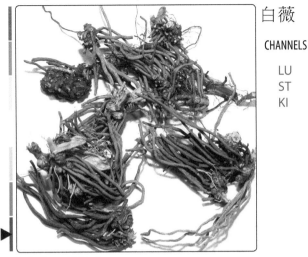

CHANNELS

LU
ST
KI

Radix Cynanchi Atrati
bitter, salty, cold

chì sháo (Red Peony Root)

赤芍

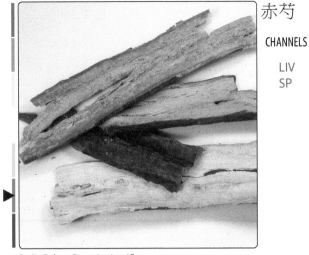

CHANNELS

LIV
SP

Radix Rubrus Paeoniae Lactiflorae
sour, bitter, slightly cold

dì gǔ pí (Cortex of Wolfberry Root or Lycium Bark)

地骨皮

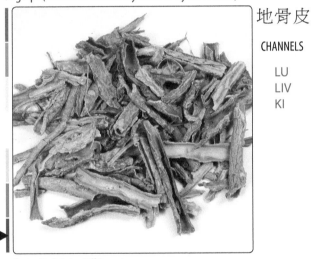

CHANNELS

LU
LIV
KI

Cortex Radicis Lycii Chinensis
sweet, cold

mǔ dān pí (Cortex of the Peony Tree Root)

牡丹皮

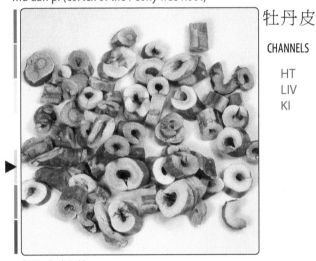

CHANNELS

HT
LIV
KI

Cortex Radicis Moutan
spicy, bitter, cool

shēng dì huáng (Chinese Foxglove Root, Rehmannia)

地黃

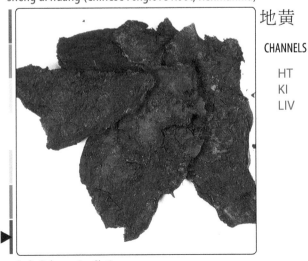

CHANNELS

HT
KI
LIV

Radix Rehmanniae Glutinosae
sweet, bitter, cold

xī jiǎo (Rhinoceros Horn)

shui niu jiao shown

犀角

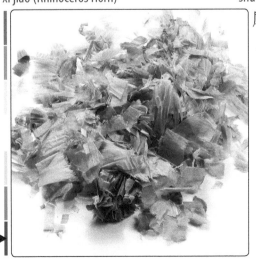

CHANNELS

HT
LIV
ST

Cornu Rhinoceri
bitter, salty, cold

Herbs that Cool the Blood

xuán shēn (Ningpo Figwort Root)

玄参

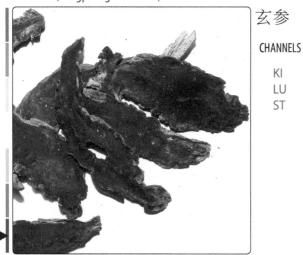

CHANNELS

KI
LU
ST

Radix Scrophulariae Ningpoensis
salty, sweet, bitter, cold

yīn chái hú (Stellaria Root)

阴柴胡

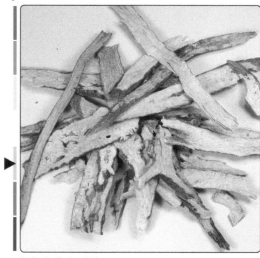

CHANNELS

LIV
ST

Radix Stellariae Dichotomae
sweet, cool

zǐ cǎo (Groomwell Root or Arnebia or Lithospermum)

紫草

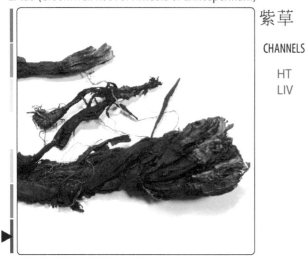

CHANNELS

HT
LIV

Radix Arnebiae seu Lithospermi
sweet, cold

hú huáng lián (Picrorhiza Rhizome)

胡簧莲

CHANNELS

LIV
ST
LI.

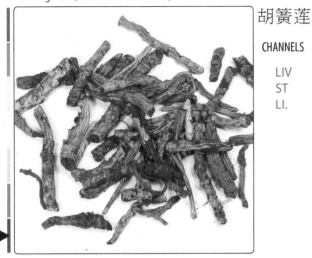

Rhizoma Picrorrhizae
bitter, cold

huáng bǎi (Phellodendron or Amur Cork tree Bark)

黄柏

CHANNELS

KI
BL

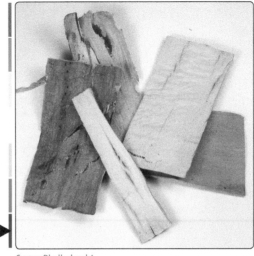

Cortex Phellodendri
bitter, cold

huáng lián (Coptis Rhizome)

黄连

CHANNELS

HT
LI
LIV
ST

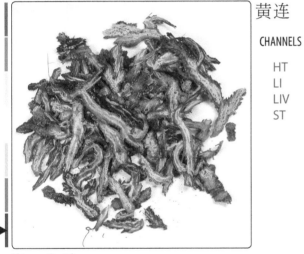

Rhizoma Coptidis
bitter, cold

huáng qín (Baical Skullcap Root)

黄芩

CHANNELS

GB
LI
LU
ST

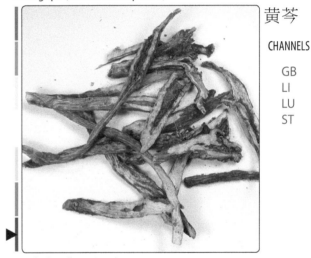

Radix Scutellariae Baicalensis
bitter, cold

kǔ shēn (Sophora Root)

苦参

CHANNELS

BL
HT
LIV
LI
SI

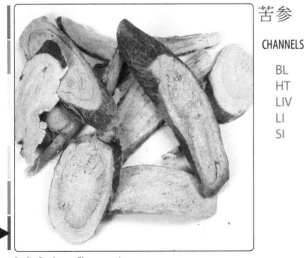

Radix Sophorae Flavescentis
bitter, cold

lóng dǎn cǎo (Chinese Gentian Root)

龙胆草

CHANNELS

GB
LIV
ST

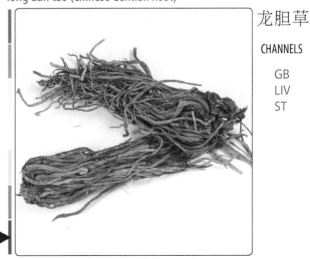

Radix Gentianae Longdancao
bitter, cold

qín pí (Korean Ash Branch Bark)

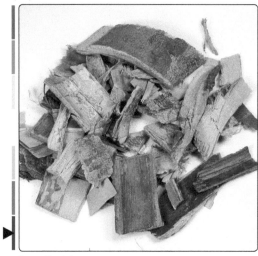

秦皮

CHANNELS

GB
LI
LIV
ST

Cortex Fraxini
bitter, cold

bái huā shé shé căo (Oldenlandia or Heydyotis)

白花蛇舌草

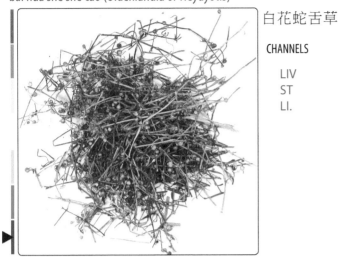

CHANNELS

LIV
ST
LI.

Herba Hedyotidis Diffusae
bitter, sweet, cold

bài jiàng căo (Patrinia, Thiaspi)

败酱草

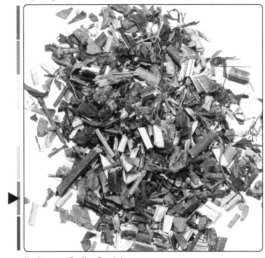

CHANNELS

LI
LIV
ST

Herba cum Radice Patriniae
spicy, bitter, slightly cold

bái tóu wēng (Chinese Anemone Root or Pulsatilla)

白头翁

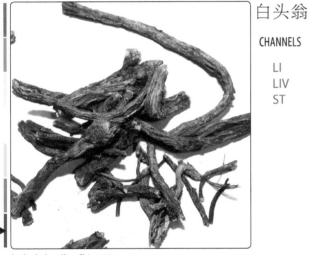

CHANNELS

LI
LIV
ST

Radix Pulsatillae Chinensis
bitter, cold

bái xiăn pí (Cortex of Chinese Dittany Root)

白鲜皮

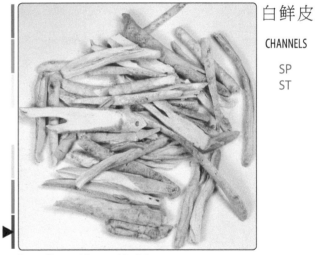

CHANNELS

SP
ST

Cortex Dictamni Dasycarpi Radicis
bitter, cold

băn lán gēn (Woad Root or Isatis Root)

板蓝根

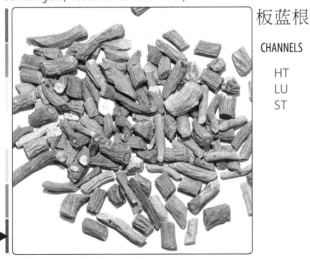

CHANNELS

HT
LU
ST

Radix Isatidis seu Baphicacanthi
bitter, cold

bàn zhī lián (Barbat Skullcap or Scutellaria)

半枝莲

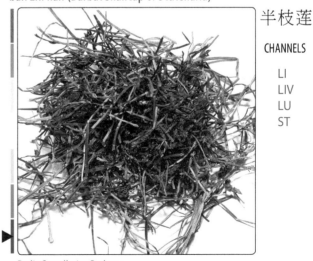

CHANNELS

LI
LIV
LU
ST

Radix Scutellariae Barbatae
spicy, bitter, cold

Herbs that Clear Heat and Eliminate Toxins

chuān xīn lián (Green Chiretta or Kariyat or Andrographis)

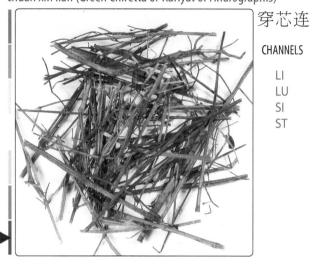

穿芯连

CHANNELS

LI
LU
SI
ST

Herba Andrographitis Paniculatae
bitter, cold

dài qīng yè (Indigo or Woad Leaf)

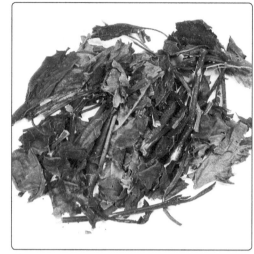

大青叶

CHANNELS

HT
LU
ST

Folium Daqingye
bitter, very cold

hóng téng (Sargentodoxa Vine)

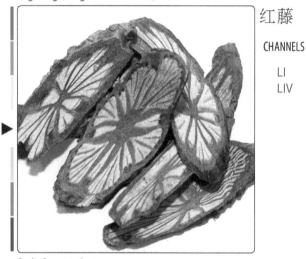

红藤

CHANNELS

LI
LIV

Caulis Sargentodoxae
bitter, neutral

jīn yín huā (Honeysuckle Flower or Lonicera)

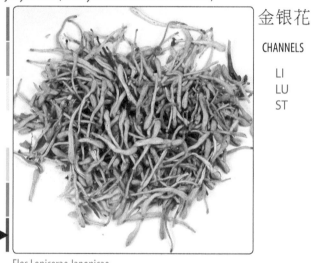

金银花

CHANNELS

LI
LU
ST

Flos Lonicerae Japonicae
sweet, cold

lián qiáo (Forsythia Fruit)

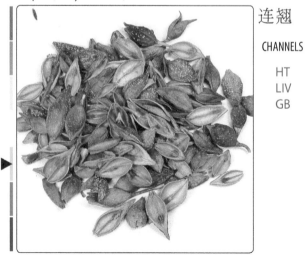

连翘

CHANNELS

HT
LIV
GB

Fructus Forsythiae Suspensae
bitter, slightly spicy, cool

lòu lú (Echinops Root or Rhaponticum)

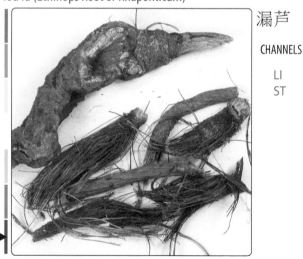

漏芦

CHANNELS

LI
ST

Radix Rhapontici seu Echinopsis
bitter, salty, cold

mǎ bó (Fruiting Body of Puffball or Lasiosphaera)

马勃

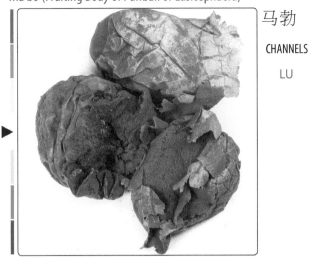

CHANNELS

LU

Fructificatio Lasiosphaerae seu Calvatiae
spicy, neutral

mǎ chǐ xiàn (Purslane or Portulaca)

马齿苋

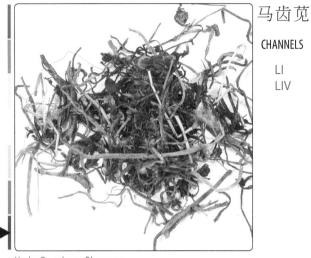

CHANNELS

LI
LIV

Herba Portulacae Oleraceae
sour, cold

pú gōng Yīng (Dandelion)

蒲公英

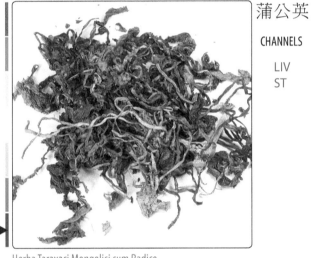

CHANNELS

LIV
ST

Herba Taraxaci Mongolici cum Radice
bitter, sweet, cold

qīng dài (Indigo)

青黛

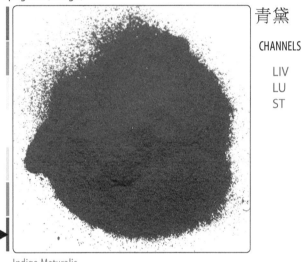

CHANNELS

LIV
LU
ST

Indigo Maturalis
salty, cold

rěn dōng téng (Honeysuckle Stem)

忍冬疼

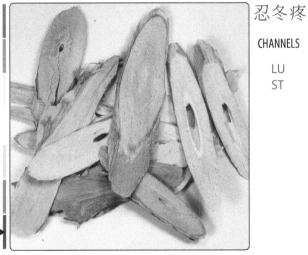

CHANNELS

LU
ST

Caulis Lonicerae
sweet, cold

shān dòu gēn (Sophora Root or Subprostrate)

山豆根

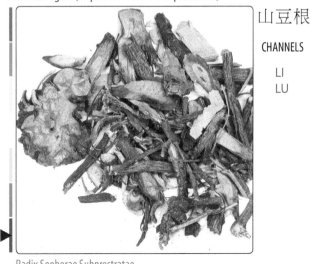

CHANNELS

LI
LU

Radix Sophorae Subprostratae
bitter, cold

Herbs that Clear Heat and Eliminate Toxins

shè gàn (Belamcanda Rhizome)

射干

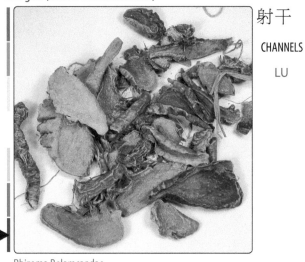

CHANNELS

LU

Rhizoma Belamcandae
bitter, cold

tǔ fú líng (Smilax or Glabrous Greenbrier Rhizome)

土茯苓

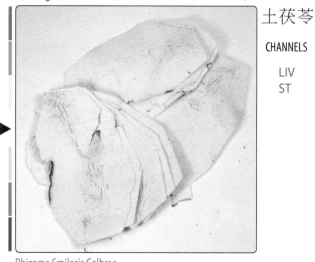

CHANNELS

LIV
ST

Rhizoma Smilacis Galbrae
sweet, bland, neutral

niú xī (Tuniuxi Root)

牛膝

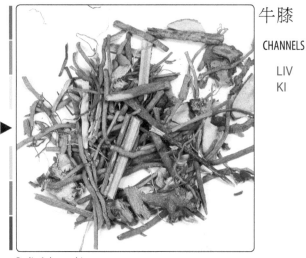

CHANNELS

LIV
KI

Radix Achyranthis
bitter, sour, neutral

yā dàn zǐ (Java Brucea Fruit)

鸭蛋子

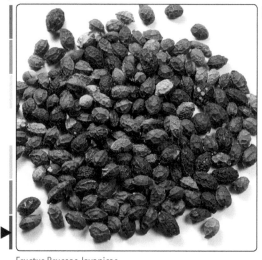

CHANNELS

LI
LIV

Fructus Bruceae Javanicae
bitter, cold ,toxic

yě jú huā (Wild Chrysanthemum Flower)

野菊花

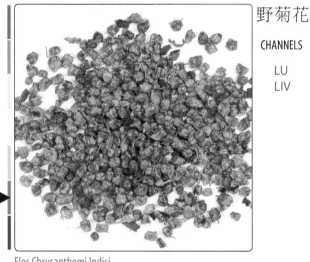

CHANNELS

LU
LIV

Flos Chrysanthemi Indici
bitter, spicy, slightly cold

yú xīng cǎo (Houttuynia)

鱼腥草

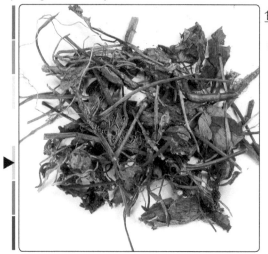

CHANNELS

LI
LU

Herba cum Radice Houttuyniae Cordatae
spicy, cool

zǐ huā dì dīng (Viola or Yedeon's Violet)

紫花地丁

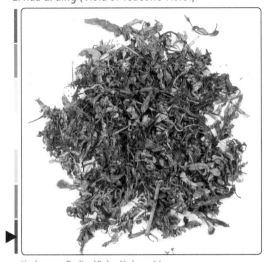

CHANNELS

HT
LIV

Herba cum Radice Violae Yedoensitis
spicy, bitter, cold

bái biăn dòu (Hyacinth Bean, Dolichos)

白扁豆

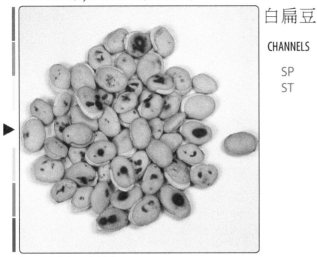

CHANNELS

SP
ST

Semen Dolichoris Lablab
sweet, neutral

dà dòu juăn (Young Soybean Sprout)

大豆卷

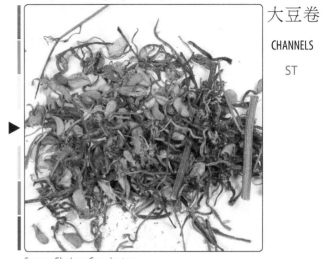

CHANNELS

ST

Semen Glycines Germinatum
sweet, neutral

hè yè (Lotus Leaf)

荷叶

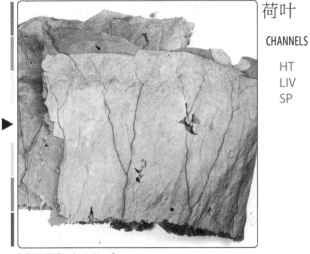

CHANNELS

HT
LIV
SP

Folium Nelumbinis Nuciferae
bitter, slightly sweet, neutral

lù dòu (Mung Bean or Phaseolus)

录豆

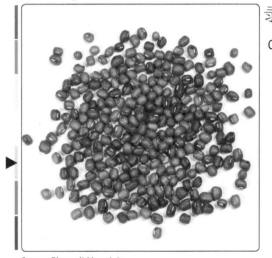

CHANNELS

HT
ST

Semen Phaseoli Munginis
sweet, cool

qīng hāo (Wormwood)

spring harvest shown

青蒿

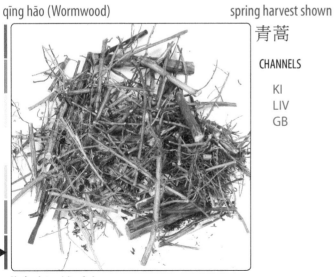

CHANNELS

KI
LIV
GB

Herba Artemisiae Apiaceae
bitter, cold

dà huáng (Rhubarb Root and Rhizome)

大簧

CHANNELS

HT
LI
LIV
ST

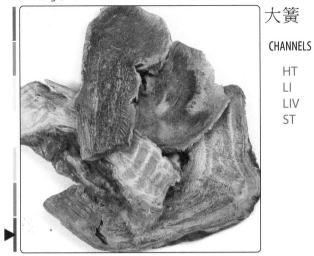

Radix Et Rhizoma Rhei
bitter, cold

fān xiè yè (Senna Leaf)

番泻叶

CHANNELS

LI.

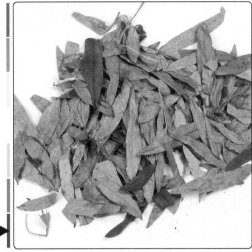

Folium Sennae
sweet, bitter, cold

máng xiāo (Sodium Sulfate, Mirabilite, Glauber's Salt)

芒硝

CHANNELS

ST
LI.

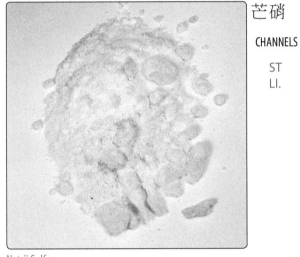

Natrii Sulfas
salty, bitter, very cold

lú huì (Aloe Leaf - Dried juice Concentrate)

芦荟

CHANNELS

LI
LIV
ST

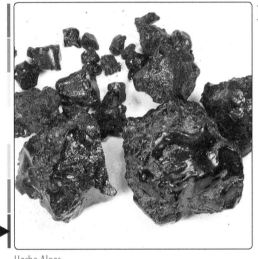

Herba Aloes
bitter, cold

huǒ má rén (Hemp Seeds or Cannabis Seeds)

火麻仁

CHANNELS

LI
SP
ST

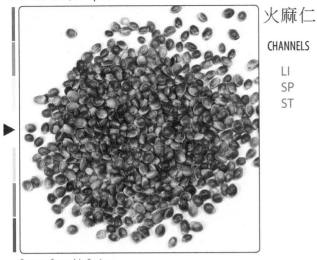

Semen Cannabis Sativae
sweet, neutral

yù lǐ rén (Bush Cherry Pit)

郁李仁

CHANNELS

LI
SI
SP

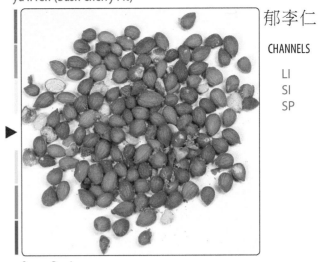

Semen Pruni
spicy, bitter, sweet, neutral

郁李仁

bā dòu (Croton Seed)

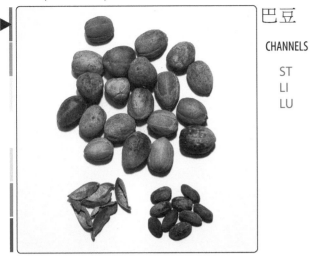

巴豆

CHANNELS

ST
LI
LU

Crotonis Fructus
spicy, hot, toxic

hóng dà jǐ (Peking Spurge Root or Euphorbia)

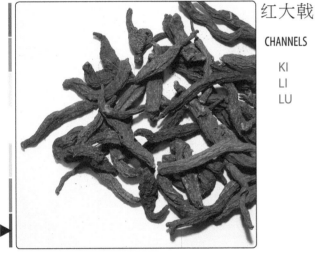

红大戟

CHANNELS

KI
LI
LU

Radix Euphorbiae seu Knoxiae
bitter, spicy, cold, toxic

yuán hu (Genkwa Flower)

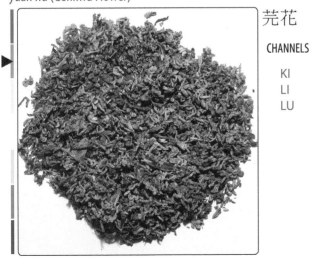

芫花

CHANNELS

KI
LI
LU

Flos Daphnis Genkwae
bitter, spicy, warm, toxic

gān suì (Kansui Root)

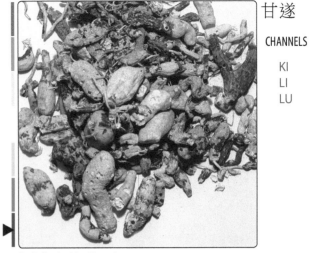

甘遂

CHANNELS

KI
LI
LU

Radix Euphorbiae Kansui
bitter, sweet, cold, toxic

Shāng lù (Poke Root or Phytolacca)

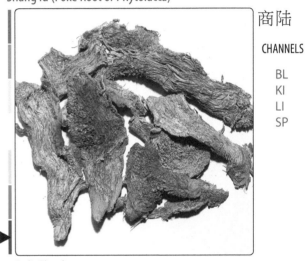

商陆

CHANNELS

BL
KI
LI
SP

Radix Phytolaccae
bitter, cold, toxic

bā yuè zhá (Akebia Fruit)

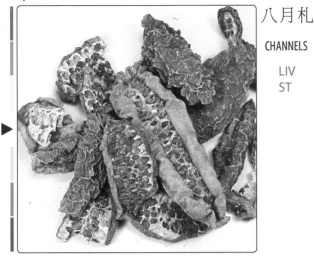

八月札

CHANNELS

LIV
ST

Fructus Akebiae Trifoliatae
bitter, neutral

bì xiè (Fish Poison Yam Rhizome, Tokoro)

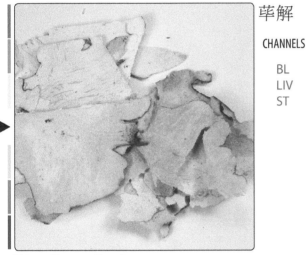

萆解

CHANNELS

BL
LIV
ST

Rhizoma Dioscoreae Hypoglaucae
bitter, neutral

chē qián zǐ (Plantago Seed, Plantain Seed)

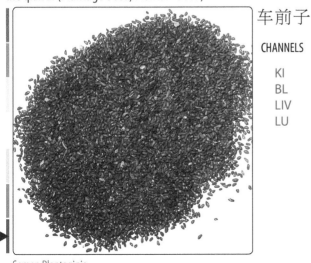

车前子

CHANNELS

KI
BL
LIV
LU

Semen Plantaginis
sweet, cold

bàn biàn lián (Chinese Lobelia, Lobelia)

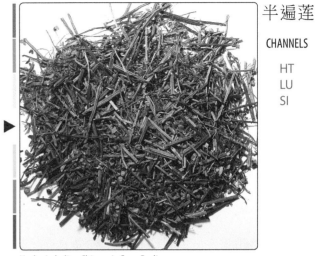

半遍莲

CHANNELS

HT
LU
SI

Herba Lobeliae Chinensis Gum Radice
sweet, neutral

biǎn xù (Knotweed, Polygonum)

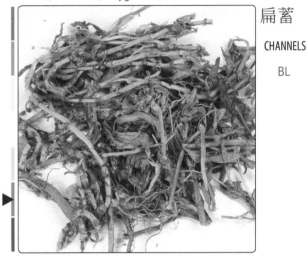

扁蓄

CHANNELS

BL

Herba Polygoni Avicularis
bitter, slightly cold

chì xiǎo dòu (Aduki Bean, Phaseolus)

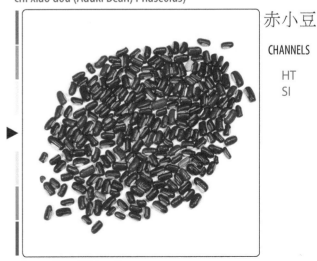

赤小豆

CHANNELS

HT
SI

Semen Phaseoli Calcarati
sweet, sour, neutral

Herbs that Regulate Water and Drain Dampness

dēng xīn cǎo (Rush Pith, Juncus)

灯心草

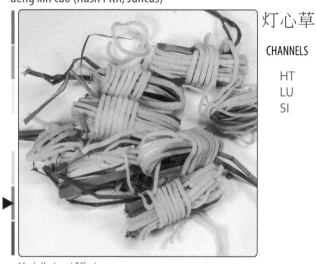

CHANNELS

HT
LU
SI

Medulla Junci Effusi
sweet, bland, slightly cold

dì fū zǐ (Broom Cypress, Kochia Fruit)

地肤子

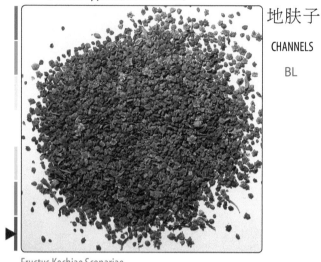

CHANNELS

BL

Fructus Kochiae Scopariae
sweet, bitter, cold

dōng guā zǐ (Winter Melon, Wax Gourd Seed, Benincasa)

冬瓜子

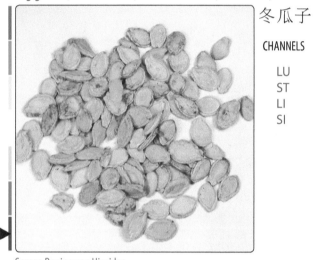

CHANNELS

LU
ST
LI
SI

Semen Benincasae Hispidae
sweet, cold

dōng kuí zǐ (Musk Mallow Seeds, Abutilon Seeds)

冬葵子

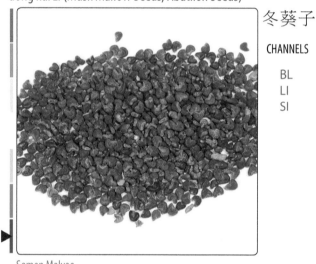

CHANNELS

BL
LI
SI

Semen Malvae
sweet, cold

fú líng (Sclerotium of Tuckahoe, China Root, Poria, Hoelen)

茯苓

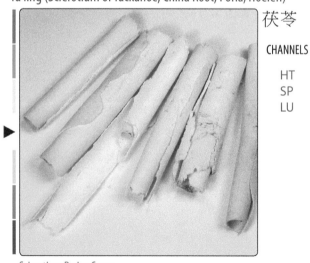

CHANNELS

HT
SP
LU

Sclerotium Poriae Cocos
sweet, bland, neutral

fú líng pí (Poria Skin)

茯苓皮

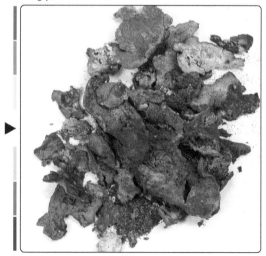

CHANNELS

HT
SP
LU

Sclerotii Poriae Cocos
sweet, bland, neutral

fú shén (Poria Spirit)

茯神

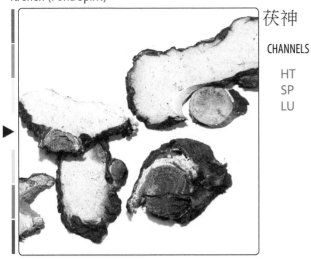

CHANNELS

HT
SP
LU

Scierotium Pararadicis Poriae Cocos
sweet, bland, neutral

hǎi Jīn shā (Spores of Japanese Fern)

海金沙

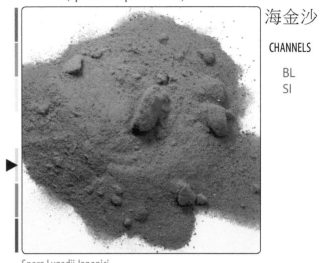

CHANNELS

BL
SI

Spora Lygodii Japonici
sweet, cool

hàn fáng jǐ (Stephania Root)

防己

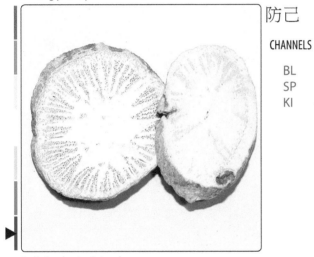

CHANNELS

BL
SP
KI

Radix Stephaniae Tetrandrae
bitter, spicy, cold

huá shí (Talcum)

滑石

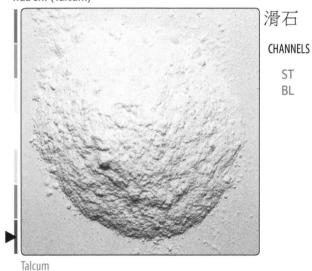

CHANNELS

ST
BL

Talcum
sweet, bland, cold

jīn qiān cǎo (Lysimachia)

金千草

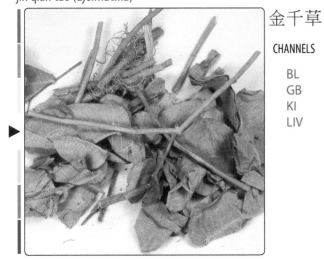

CHANNELS

BL
GB
KI
LIV

Herba Desmodii Styrachifolii
sweet, bland, neutral

chuān mù tōng (Clematis)

木通

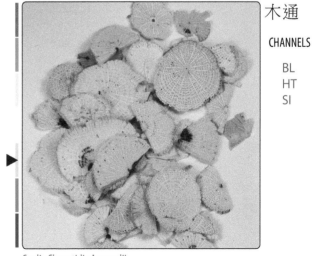

CHANNELS

BL
HT
SI

Caulis Clematidis Armandii
bitter, cool

Herbs that Regulate Water and Drain Dampness

qú mài (Aerial Parts of Fringed Pink or Chinese Pink Dianthus)

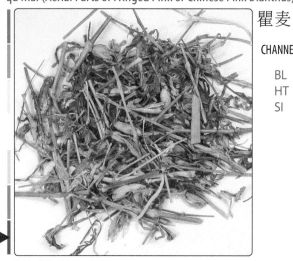

瞿麦

CHANNELS

BL
HT
SI

Herba Dianthi
bitter, cold

shí wěi (Pyrrosia Leaves)

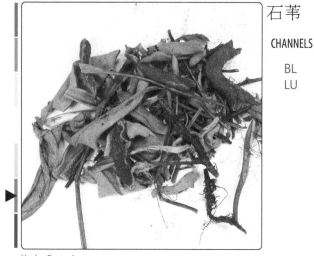

石苇

CHANNELS

BL
LU

Herba Pyrrosiae
bitter, sweet, slightly cold

tōng cǎo (Rice Paper Pith, Tetrapanax)

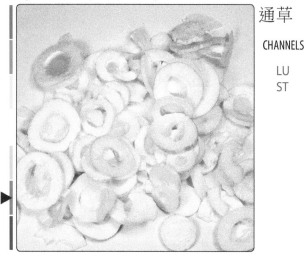

通草

CHANNELS

LU
ST

Medulla Tetrapanacis Papyriferi
sweet, bland, slightly cold

yì yǐ rén (Seeds of Job's Tears)

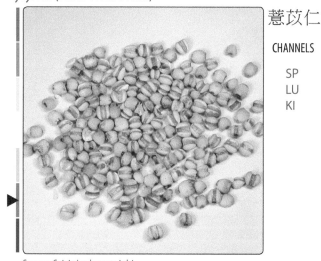

薏苡仁

CHANNELS

SP
LU
KI

Semen Coicis Lachyrma-jobi
sweet, bland, slightly cold

yīn chén (Yinchenhao Shoots and Leaves, Capillaris)

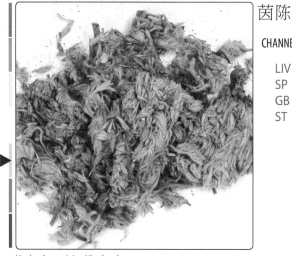

茵陈

CHANNELS

LIV
SP
GB
ST

Herba Artemisiae Yinchenhao
bitter, spicy, cool

yù mǐ xū (Cornsilk)

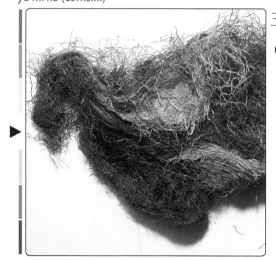

玉米须

CHANNELS

BL
GB
LIV

Stylus Zeae Mays
sweet, neutral

zé xiè (Water Plantain Rhizome, Alisma)

泽泻

CHANNELS

KI
BL

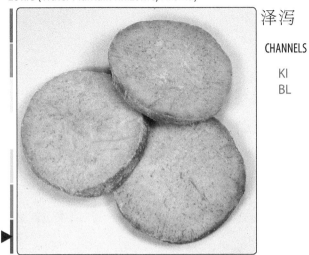

Rhizoma Alismatis
sweet, bland, cold

zhū líng (Polyporus Sclerotium)

猪苓

CHANNELS

SP
KI
BL

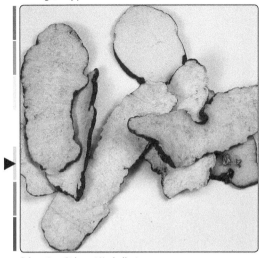

Sclerotium Polypori Umbellati
sweet, bland, cool (or neutral)

泽泻 猪苓

cán shā (Silkworm Feces)

蚕沙

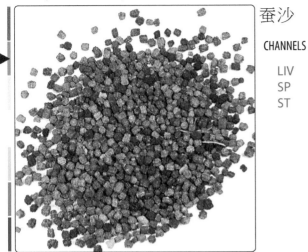

CHANNELS

LIV
SP
ST

Excrementum Bombycis Mon
sweet, spicy, warm

cāng ěr zǐ (Cocklebur Fruit)

苍耳子

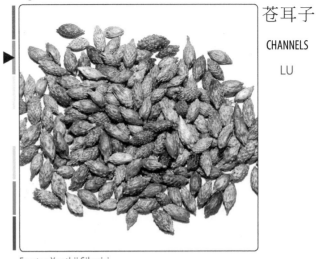

CHANNELS

LU

Fructus Xanthii Siberici
sweet, bitter, warm, toxic

dú huó (Pubescent Angelica Root)

独活

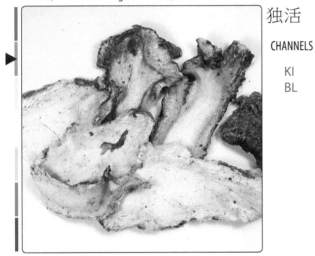

CHANNELS

KI
BL

Radix Angelicae Pubescentis
bitter, spicy, warm

hǎi fēng téng (Kadsura Stem)

海风藤

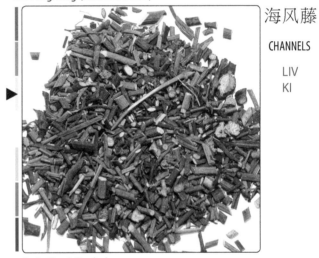

CHANNELS

LIV
KI

Caulis Piperis Futokadsurae
spicy, bitter, slightly warm

hǎi tóng pí (Coral Bean Back)

海桐皮

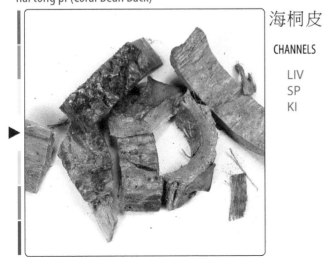

CHANNELS

LIV
SP
KI

Cortex Erythriniae
bitter, spicy, neutral

hǔ gǔ (Tiger Bone)

虎骨

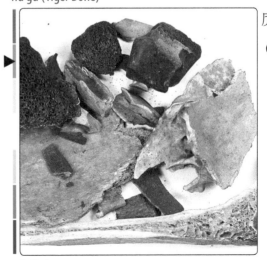

CHANNELS

LIV
KI

Os Tigris
spicy, sweet, warm

kuān jīn téng (Chinese Tinospora Stem)

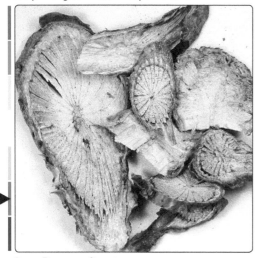

CHANNELS

LIV

Ramus Tinosporae Sinensis
bitter, slightly cold

luò shí téng (Star Jasmine Stem)

络石藤

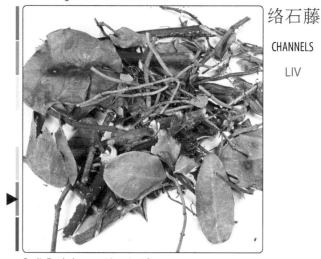

CHANNELS

LIV

Caulis Trachelospermi Jasminoidis
bitter, slightly cold

mù guā (Chinese Quince Fruit)

木瓜

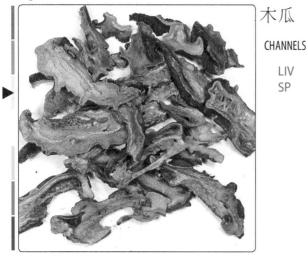

CHANNELS

LIV
SP

Fructus Chaenomelis Lagenariae
sour, slightly warm

qiān nián jiàn (Homalomena Rhizome)

千年健

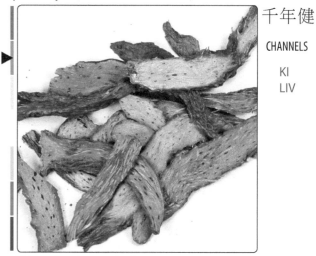

CHANNELS

KI
LIV

Rhizoma Homalomenae Occultae
spicy, bitter, warm

qín jiāo (Gentiana Macrophylla Root)

秦艽

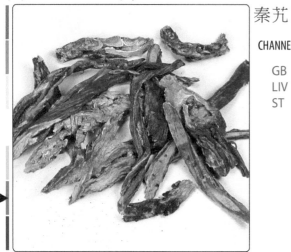

CHANNELS

GB
LIV
ST

Radix Gentianae Macrophyllae
bitter, spicy, slightly cold

sāng zhī (Mulberry Twig)

桑枝

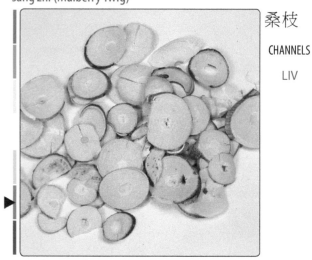

CHANNELS

LIV

Ramulus Mori Albae
bitter, sweet, slightly cold

wēi líng xiān (Chinese Clematis Root)

威灵仙

CHANNELS

BL

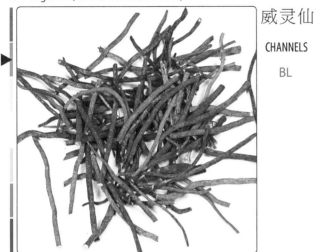

Radix Clematidis Chinensis
spicy, salty, warm

wǔ jiā pí (Acanthopanax Root Bark)

五加皮

CHANNELS

KI
LIV

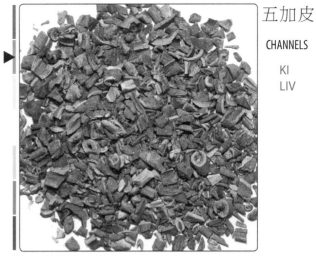

Cortex Radicis Acanthopanacis Gracistyli
spicy, bitter, warm

xī xiān cǎo (Siegesbeckia)

希莶草

CHANNELS

KI
LIV

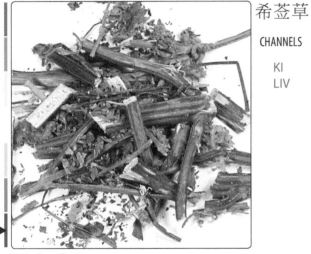

Herba Siegesbeckiae
bitter, cold

chuān bèi mǔ (Tendrilled Fritillaria Bulb)

川贝母

CHANNELS

HT
LU

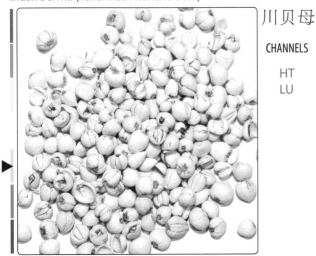

Bulbus Fritillariae Cirrhosae
bitter, sweet, cool

dǎn nán xīng (Jack-in-the-Pulpit Rhizome & Bile)

胆南星

CHANNELS

LIV
LU
SP

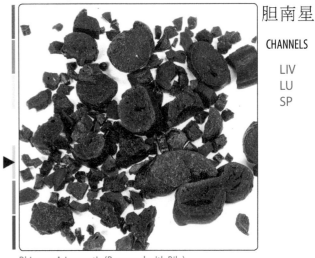

Rhizoma Arisaematis (Processed with Bile)
bitter, cool

fú hǎi shí (Pumice)

浮海石

CHANNELS

LU

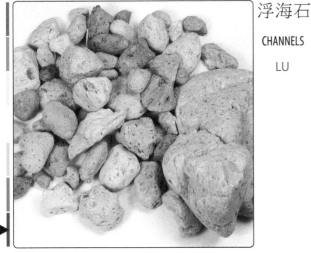

Pumice
salty, cold

guā lóu (Trichosanthes Fruit)

栝楼

CHANNELS

LI
LU
ST

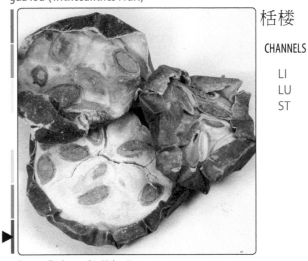

Fructus Trichosanthis Kirlowii
sweet, cold

guā lóu pí (Trichosanthes Peel, Snake Gourd Peel)

栝楼皮

CHANNELS

LI
LU
ST

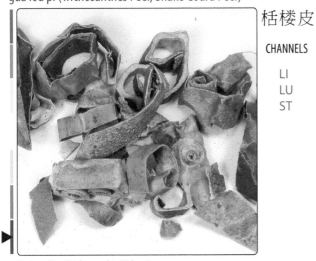

Pericarpium Trichosanthis Kirlowii
sweet, cold

guā lóu rén (Trichosanthes Seeds)

栝楼仁

CHANNELS

LI
LU
ST

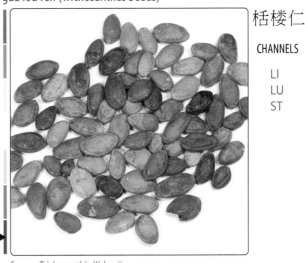

Semen Trichosanthis Kirlowii
sweet, cold

hǎi zǎo (Seaweed, Sargassum)

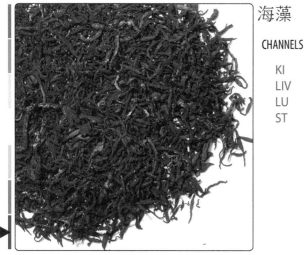

海藻

CHANNELS

KI
LIV
LU
ST

Herba Sargassii
bitter, salty, cold

huáng yào zǐ (Dioscorea Bulbifera Tober)

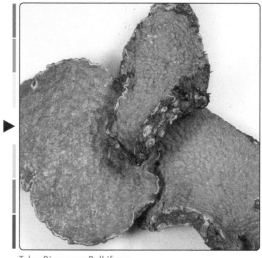

CHANNELS

HT
LIV
LU

Tuber Dioscoreae Bulbiferae
bitter, neutral

kūn bù (Kelp, Eckloniae Thallus)

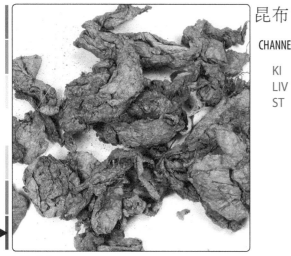

昆布

CHANNELS

KI
LIV
ST

Ecklonia Kurome
salty, cold

pàng dà hǎi (Boat Sterculia Seed)

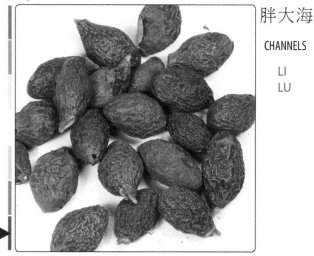

胖大海

CHANNELS

LI
LU

Sterculiae lychnophorae Semen
sweet, cold

qián hú (Hogfennel Root)

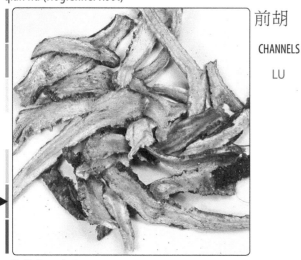

前胡

CHANNELS

LU

Radix Peucedani
bitter, spicy, slightly cold

tiān huā fēn (Trichosanthes Root)

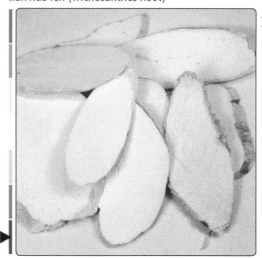

天花分

CHANNELS

LU
ST

Trichosanthis Kirlowii Radix
bitter, slightly sweet, cold

tiān zhú huáng (Siliceous Secretions of Bamboo, Tabasheer)

天竺黄

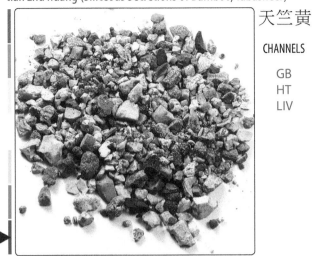

Bambusae Concretio Silicea
sweet, cold

CHANNELS

GB
HT
LIV

Zhè bèi mǔ (Thunberg Fritillaria Bulb)

浙贝母

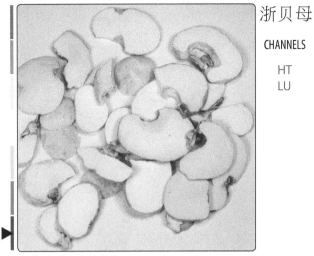

Fritillariae Thunbergii Bulbus
bitter, cold

CHANNELS

HT
LU

zhú rù (Bamboo Shavings)

竹茹

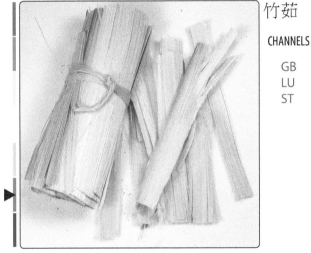

Bambusae Caulis In Taeniam
sweet, slightly cold

CHANNELS

GB
LU
ST

bái fù zǐ (Typhonium Rhizome)

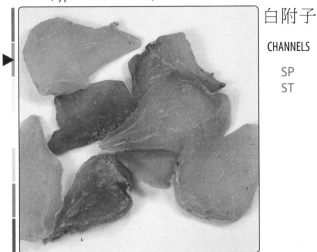

白附子

CHANNELS

SP
ST

Rhizoma Typhonii Gigantei
spicy, sweet, warm, toxic

bái jiè zǐ (White Mustard Seed)

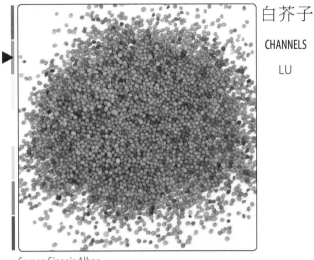

白芥子

CHANNELS

LU

Semen Sinapis Albae
spicy, warm

bái qián (Root and Rhizome of Cynanchum)

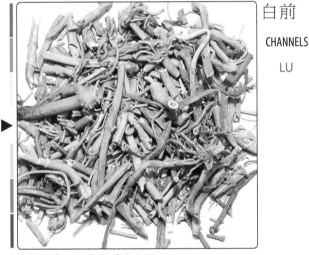

白前

CHANNELS

LU

Radix Et Rhizoma Cynanchi Baiqian
spicy, sweet, neutral (or slightly warm)

bàn xià (Pinellia Rhizome)

sheng ban xia shown

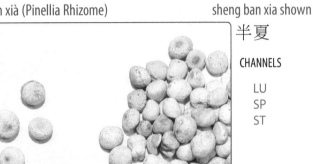

半夏

CHANNELS

LU
SP
ST

Rhizoma Pinelliae Tematae
spicy, warm, toxic

jié gěng (Root of the Balloon Flower)

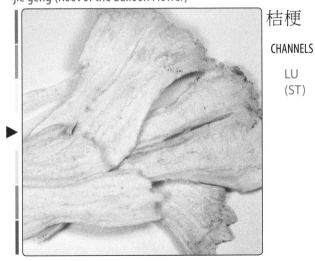

桔梗

CHANNELS

LU
(ST)

Platycodi Radix
bitter, spicy, neutral

xuàn fù huā (Inula Flower)

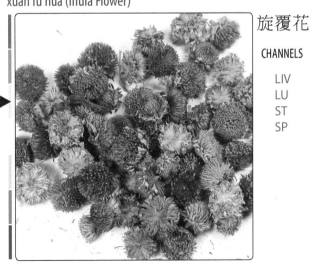

旋覆花

CHANNELS

LIV
LU
ST
SP

Inulae Flos
bitter, spicy, slightly warm

zào jiǎo cì (Spine of Chinese Honeylocust Fruit)

皂角刺

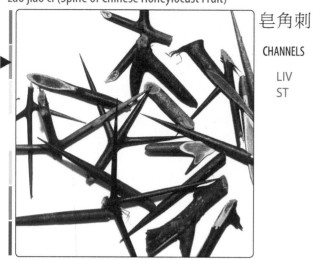

CHANNELS

LIV
ST

Gleditschiae Sinensis Spina
spicy, warm

zhì tiān nán xīng (Prepared Jack in the Pulpit Rhizome)

制天南星

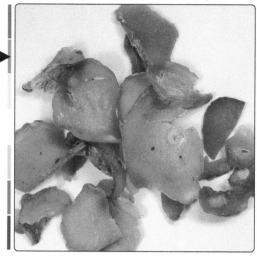

CHANNELS

LIV
LU
SP

Arisaematis Rhizoma preparatum
bitter, spicy, warm, toxic

bǎi bù (Stemona Root)

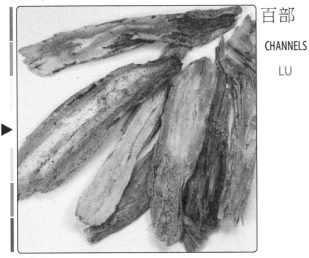

百部

CHANNELS

LU

Radix Stemonae
sweet, bitter, slightly warm (or neutral)

mǎ dōu líng (Birthwort Fruit)

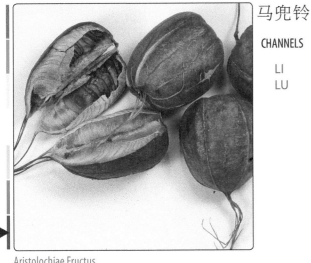

马兜铃

CHANNELS

LI
LU

Aristolochiae Fructus
bitter, slightly spicy, cold, toxic

pí pa yè (Loquat Leaf)

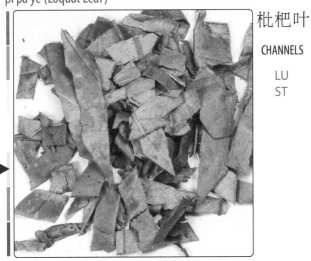

枇杷叶

CHANNELS

LU
ST

Folium Eriobotryae Japonicae
bitter, cool

kuǎn dōng huā (Coltsfoot Flower)

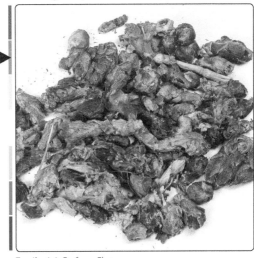

款冬花

CHANNELS

LU

Tussilaginis Farfarae Flos
spicy, warm

mù hú dié (Oroxylum Seeds)

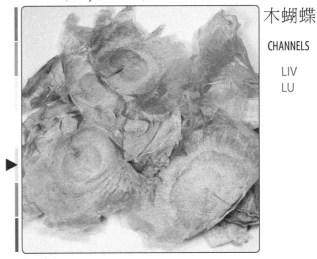

木蝴蝶

CHANNELS

LIV
LU

Oroxyli Semen
sweet, bland, cool

sāng bái pí (Bark of Mulberry Root)

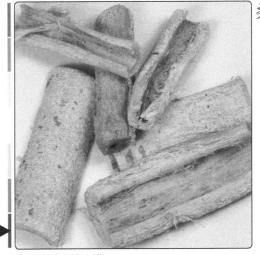

桑白皮

CHANNELS

LU
SP

Cortex Radicis Mori Albae
sweet, cold

Herbs that Relieve Coughing and Wheezing

tíng lì zǐ (Descurainia Seeds)

葶苈子

CHANNELS

LU
BL

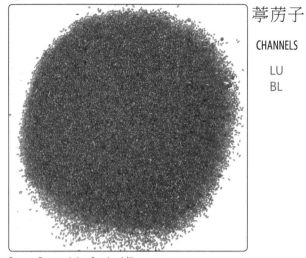

Semen Descurainiae Seu Lepidii
spicy, bitter, very cold

xìng rén (Apricot Seed or Kernel)

杏仁

CHANNELS

LI
LU

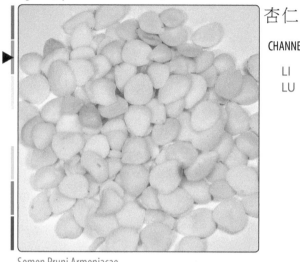

Semen Pruni Armeniacae
bitter, slightly warm, slightly toxic

zǐ sū zǐ (Purple Perilla Fruit, Perilla Seed)

紫苏子

CHANNELS

LI
LU

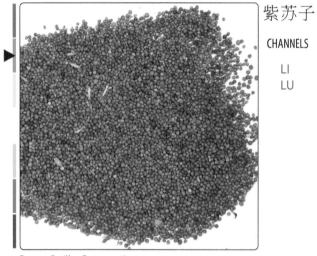

Fructus Perillae Frutescentis
spicy, warm

zǐ wǎn (Purple Aster Root)

紫菀

CHANNELS

LU

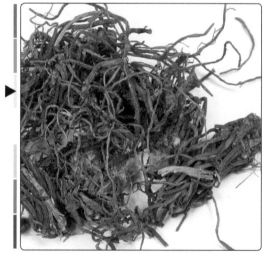

Radix Asteris Tatarici
bitter, slightly warm, sweet

bái dòu kòu (Round Cardamom Fruit)

白豆蔻

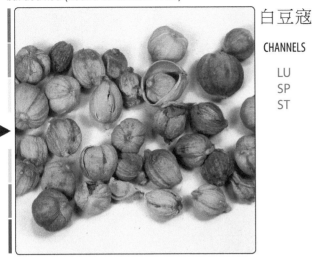

CHANNELS

LU
SP
ST

Fructus Amomi Kravanh
spicy, aromatic slightly warm (or neutral)

cǎo dòu kòu (Katsumada's Galangal Seeds)

草豆蔻

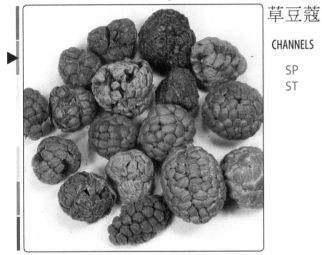

CHANNELS

SP
ST

Semen Alpiniae Katsumadai
spicy, warm, aromatic

hòu pò (Magnolia Bark)

厚朴

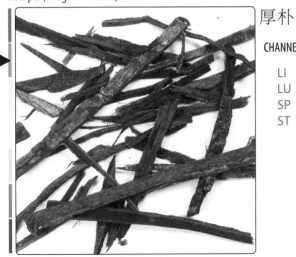

CHANNELS

LI
LU
SP
ST

Cortex Magnoliae Officinalis
bitter, spicy, warm, aromatic

cāng zhú (Black Atractylodes Rhizone)

苍术

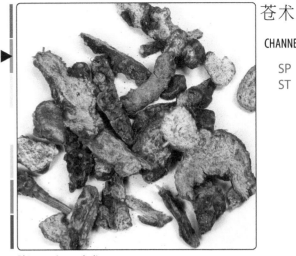

CHANNELS

SP
ST

Rhizoma Atractylodis
spicy, bitter, warm, aromatic

cǎo guǒ (Tsaoko Fruit)

草果

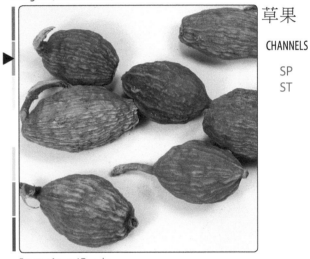

CHANNELS

SP
ST

Fructus Amomi Tsao-ko
spicy, warm

huò xiāng (Patchouli, Agastache)

藿香

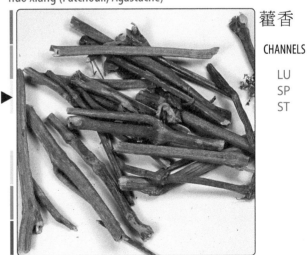

CHANNELS

LU
SP
ST

Herba Agastaches Rugosus, Herba Pogostemonis
spicy, slightly warm

pèi lán (Eupatorium)

佩兰

CHANNELS

SP
ST

Herba Eupatorii Fortunei
spicy, neutral

shā rén (Cardamom (Grains of Paradise Fruit))

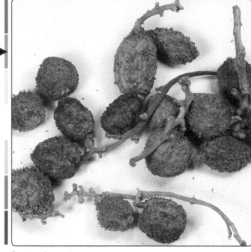

砂仁

CHANNELS

SP
ST

Fructus Amomi
spicy, warm, aromatic

gŭ yá (Rice Sprout)

谷芽

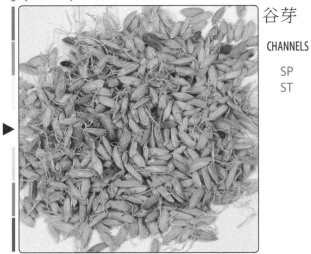

CHANNELS

SP
ST

Fructus Germinatus Oryzae Sativae
sweet, neutral

jī nèi jīn (Chicken Gizzard's Internal Lining)

鸡内金

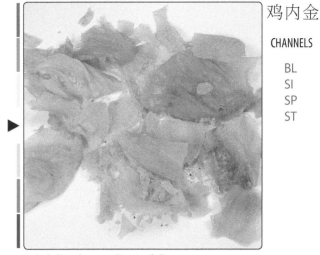

CHANNELS

BL
SI
SP
ST

Endothelium Comeum Gigeriae Galli
sweet, neutral

lái fú zǐ (Daikon, Radish Seed)

莱菔子

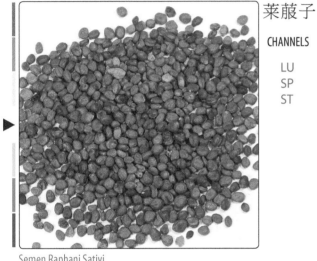

CHANNELS

LU
SP
ST

Semen Raphani Sativi
spicy, sweet, neutral

mài yá (Barley Sprout, Malt)

麦芽

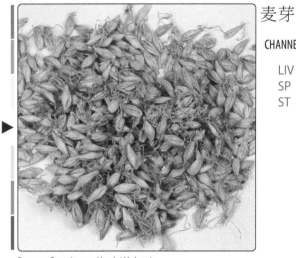

CHANNELS

LIV
SP
ST

Fructus Germinatus Hordei Vulgaris
sweet, neutral

shān zhā (Hawthorn Fruit)

山楂

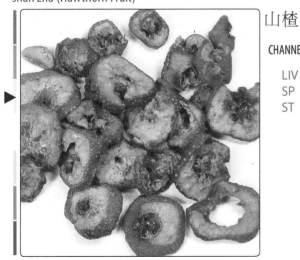

CHANNELS

LIV
SP
ST

Fructus Crataegi
sour, sweet, slightly warm

shén qǔ (Medicated Leaven)

神曲

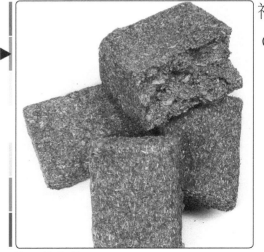

CHANNELS

SP
ST

Massa Medica Fermentata
sweet, spicy, warm

DO NOT DUPLICATE

chén pí (Orange Peel, Citrus Peel, Tangerine Peel)

陈皮

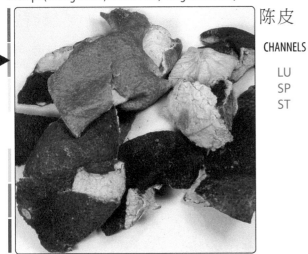

CHANNELS

LU
SP
ST

Pericarpium Citri Reticulatae
spicy, bitter, warm, aromatic

chén xiāng (Aloeswood, Aquilaria)

沉香

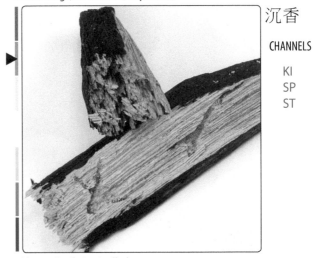

CHANNELS

KI
SP
ST

Lignum Aquilariae Agallochae
spicy, bitter, warm

chuān liàn zǐ (Sichuan Pagoda Tree Fruit)

川楝子

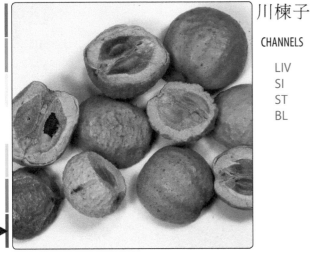

CHANNELS

LIV
SI
ST
BL

Fructus Meliae Toosendan
bitter, cold, slightly toxic

dà fù pí (Betel Husk)

大腹皮

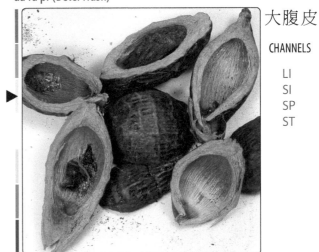

CHANNELS

LI
SI
SP
ST

Pericarpium Arecae Catechu
spicy, slightly warm

fó shǒu (Finger Citron Fruit)

佛手

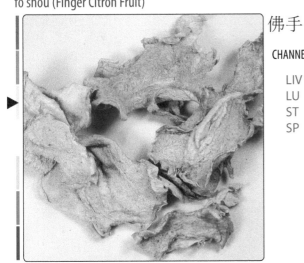

CHANNELS

LIV
LU
ST
SP

Fructus Citri Sacrodactylis
spicy, bitter, slightly warm

ju he (Citrus/Tangerine Seeds)

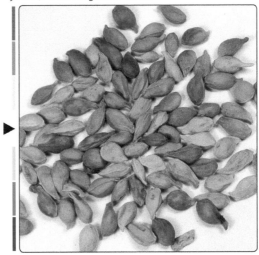

Semen Citri Reticulatae
bitter, neutral

jú hóng (Outermost Citrus Peel, Tangerine Peel, Orange Peel)

橘红

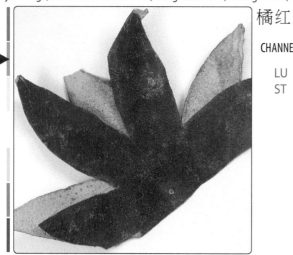

CHANNELS

LU
ST

Exocarpium Citri Rubrum
spicy, bitter, warm

lì zhī hé (Leechee Nut)

荔枝核

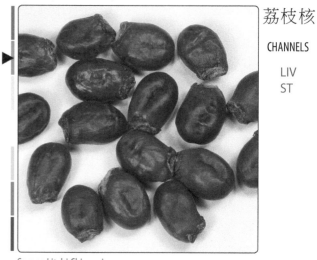

CHANNELS

LIV
ST

Semen Litchi Chinensis
sweet, astringent, warm

méi guī huā (Young Flower of Chinese Rose (Bud))

玫瑰花

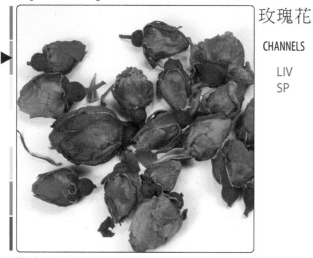

CHANNELS

LIV
SP

Flos Rosae Rugosae
sweet, slightly bitter, warm

mù xiāng (Costus Root, Saussurea)

木香

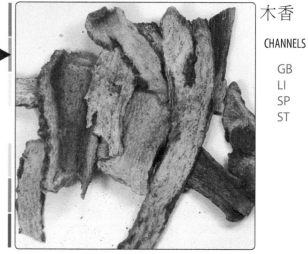

CHANNELS

GB
LI
SP
ST

Radix Auklandiae Lappae
spicy, bitter, warm

qīng pí (Immature Tangerine Peel)

青皮

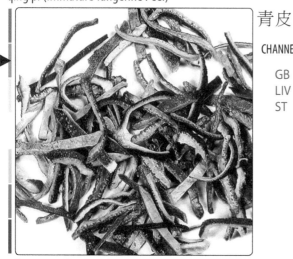

CHANNELS

GB
LIV
ST

Pericarpium Citri Reticulatae Viride
bitter, spicy, warm

shì dì (Persimmon Calyx)

柿蒂

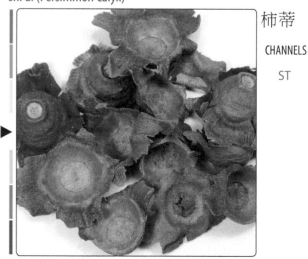

CHANNELS

ST

Calyx Diospyri Kaki
bitter, astringent, neutral

tán xiāng (Sandalwood (Heartwood))

檀香

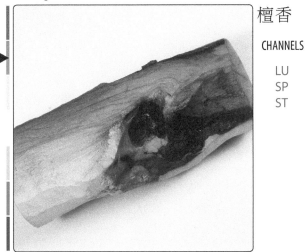

CHANNELS

LU
SP
ST

Lignum Santali Albi
spicy, warm, aromatic

wū yào (Lindera Root)

乌药

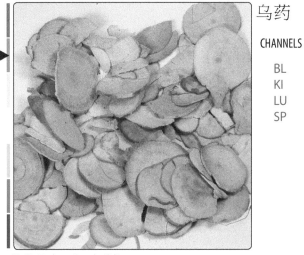

CHANNELS

BL
KI
LU
SP

Radix Linderae Strychnifoliae
spicy, warm

xiāng fù (Nut Grass Rhizome)

香附

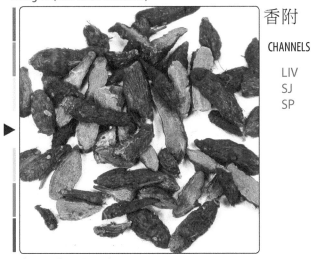

CHANNELS

LIV
SJ
SP

Rhizoma Cyperi Rotundi
spicy, slightly warm, slightly sweet, neutral

xiè bái (Bulb of Chinese Chive)

薤白

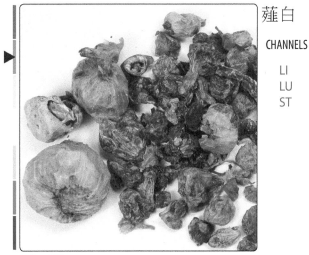

CHANNELS

LI
LU
ST

Bulbus Allii
spicy, bitter, warm

zhǐ ké (Bitter Orange Peel)

枳壳

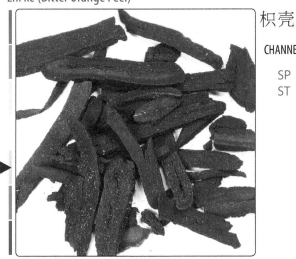

CHANNELS

SP
ST

Fructus Citri Aurantii
bitter, cool

zhǐ shí (Immature Fruit of the Bitter Orange)

枳实

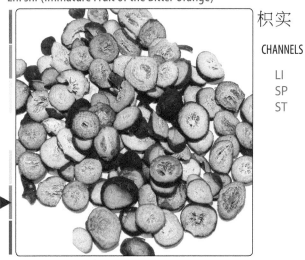

CHANNELS

LI
SP
ST

Fructus Immaturus Citri Aurantii
bitter, spicy, slightly cold

ài yè (Mugwort Leaf, Artemisia)

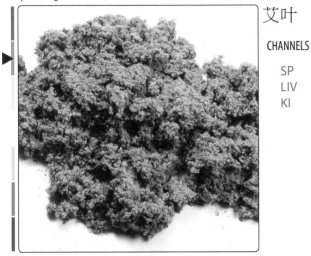

艾叶

CHANNELS

SP
LIV
KI

Artemisiae Argyi Folium
bitter, spicy, warm

bái jí (Bletilla Rhizome)

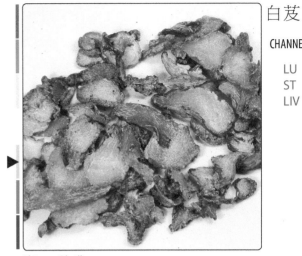

白芨

CHANNELS

LU
ST
LIV

Rhizoma Bletillae
bitter, sweet, cool, astringent

bái máo gēn (Woolly Grass Rhizome)

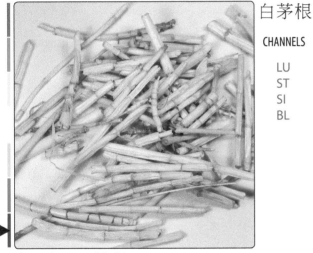

白茅根

CHANNELS

LU
ST
SI
BL

Rhizoma Imperatae Cylindricae
sweet, cold

cè bǎi yè (Biota Leaves, Leafy Twig of Arborvitae)

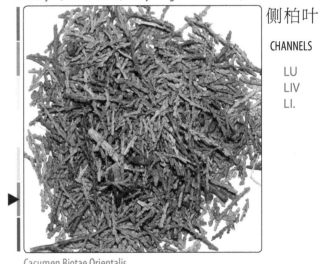

侧柏叶

CHANNELS

LU
LIV
LI.

Cacumen Biotae Orientalis
bitter, astringent, slightly cold

dài jì (Japanese Thistle, Cirsium)

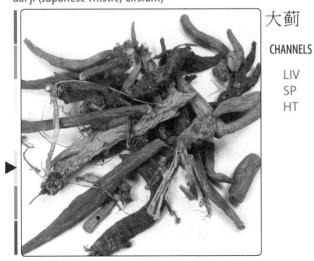

大蓟

CHANNELS

LIV
SP
HT

Herba Cirsii Japonici
sweet, cool

dì yú (Burnet Bloodwort Root)

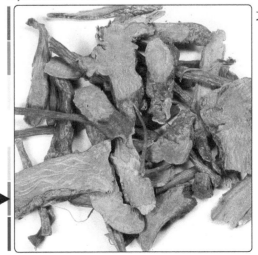

地榆

CHANNELS

LIV
LI
ST

Radix Sanguisorbae
bitter, sour, slightly cold

Herbs that Stop Bleeding

fú lóng gān (Ignited Yellow Earth)

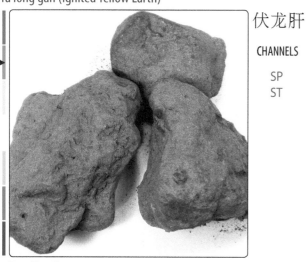

伏龙肝

CHANNELS

SP
ST

Terra Flava Usta
spicy, warm

huā ruǐ shí (Ophicalcite)

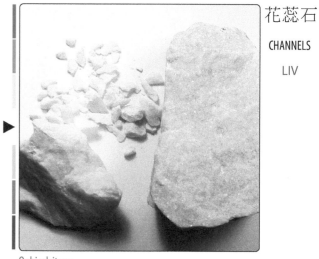

花蕊石

CHANNELS

LIV

Ophicalcitum
sour, astringent, neutral

huái huā mǐ (Pagoda Tree Flower Bud)

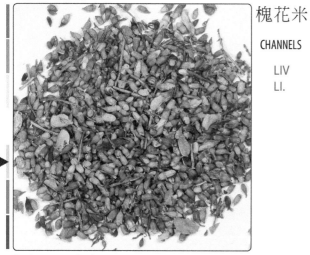

槐花米

CHANNELS

LIV
LI.

Flos Immaturus Sophorae Japonicae
bitter, cool

ŏu jié (Node of the Lotus Rhizome)

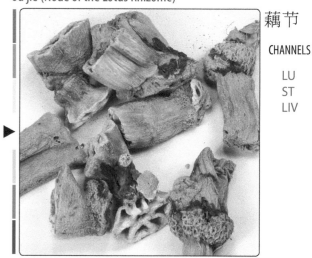

藕节

CHANNELS

LU
ST
LIV

Nodus Rhizomatis Nelumbinis Nuciferae
sweet, astringent, neutral

pú huáng (Catail Pollen)

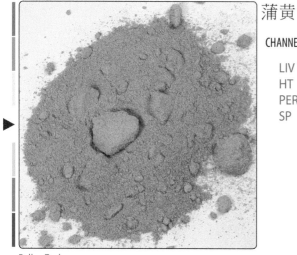

蒲黄

CHANNELS

LIV
HT
PER
SP

Pollen Typhae
sweet, spicy, neutral

qiàn cǎo (Madder Root, Rubia Root)

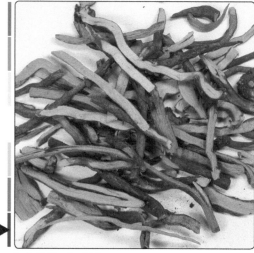

茜草

CHANNELS

HT
LIV

Radix Rubiae Cordifoliae
bitter, cold

sān qī (Notoginseng Root, Pseudoginseng Root)

三七

CHANNELS

LIV
ST
LI.

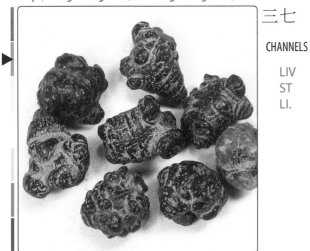

Radix Pseudoginseng
sweet, slightly bitter, warm

xiān hè cǎo (Agrimony)

仙鹤草

CHANNELS

LU
LIV
SP

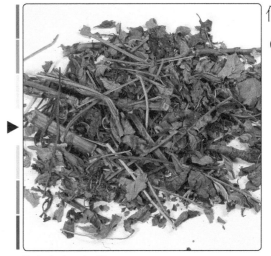

Herba Agrimoniae Pilosac
bitter, spicy, neutral

xiě yú tàn (Charred Human Hair)

血余炭

CHANNELS

HT
LIV
KI

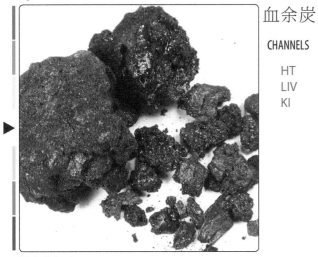

Crinis Carbonisatus
bitter, neutral

chuān niú xī (Cyathula Root)

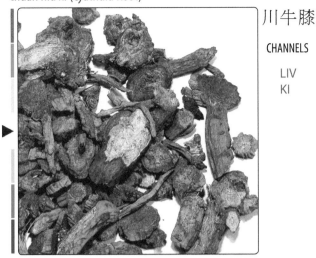

川牛膝

CHANNELS

LIV
KI

Radix Cyathula Officinalis
bitter, sour, neutral

chuān xiōng (Szechuan Lovage Root)

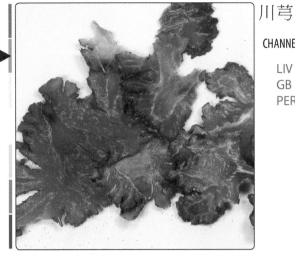

川芎

CHANNELS

LIV
GB
PER

Rhizoma Ligustici Chuanxiong
spicy, warm

dān shēn (Salvia Root)

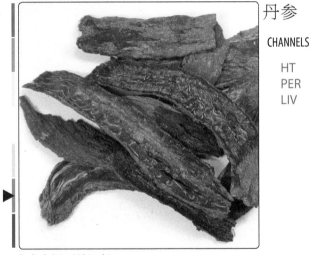

丹参

CHANNELS

HT
PER
LIV

Radix Salviae Miltiorrhizae
bitter, slightly cold

é zhú (Zedoary Rhizome)

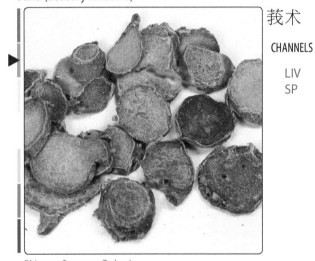

莪术

CHANNELS

LIV
SP

Rhizoma Curcumae Zedoariae
bitter, spicy, warm

hóng huā (Safflower Flower)

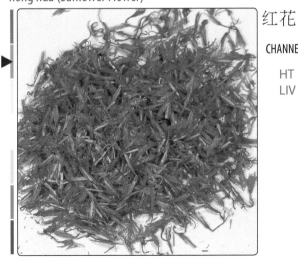

红花

CHANNELS

HT
LIV

Flos Carthami Tinctorii
spicy, warm

hǔ zhàng (Bushy Knotweed Root and Rhizome)

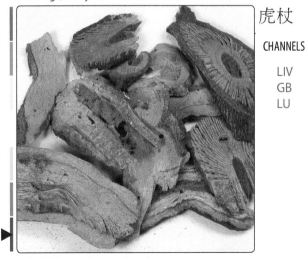

虎杖

CHANNELS

LIV
GB
LU

Radix Et Rhizoma Polygoni Cuspidati
bitter, cold

Herbs that Invigorate Blood and Remove Stagnation

huái niú xī (Achyranthes Root)
懷牛膝

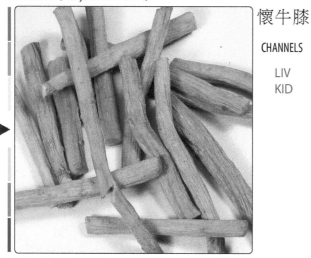

CHANNELS

LIV
KID

Radix Achyranthis Bidentatae
bitter, sour, neutral

jī xiě téng (Spatholobus, Millettia Root and Vine)
鸡血藤

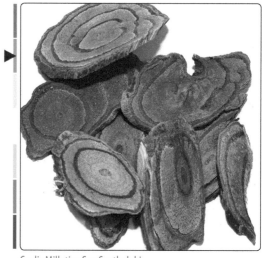

CHANNELS

HT
LIV
SP

Caulis Milletiae Seu Spatholobi
bitter, sweet, warm

jiāng huáng (Tumeric Rhizome)
姜黄

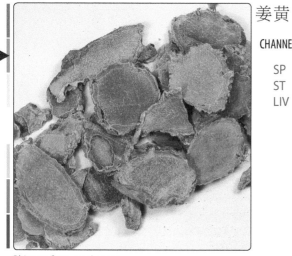

CHANNELS

SP
ST
LIV

Rhizoma Curcumae Longae
spicy, bitter, warm

Liú jì (Artemesia)
刘寄

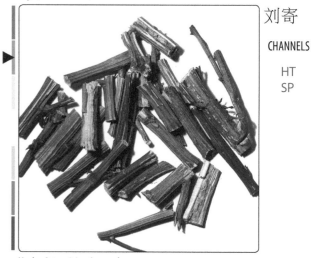

CHANNELS

HT
SP

Herba Artemisiae Anomalae
bitter, warm

lù lù tōng (Sweetgum Fruit)
路路通

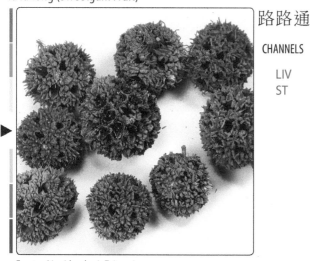

CHANNELS

LIV
ST

Fructus Liquidambaris Taiwaniae
bitter, neutral

mò yào (Myrrh)
没药

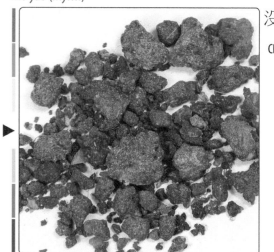

CHANNELS

HT
LIV
SP

Resina Myrrhae
bitter, neutral

rǔ xiāng (Frankincense Resin)

乳香

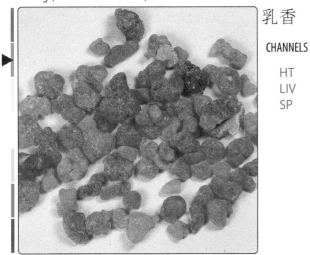

CHANNELS

HT
LIV
SP

Resina Olibani
spicy, bitter, warm

sān léng (Bur Reed Rhizome)

三棱

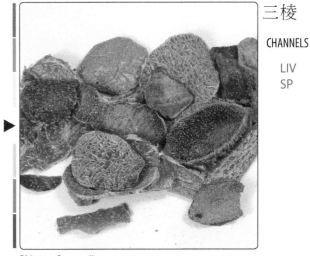

CHANNELS

LIV
SP

Rhizoma Sparganii
bitter, spicy, neutral

shuǐ zhì (Leech)

水蛭

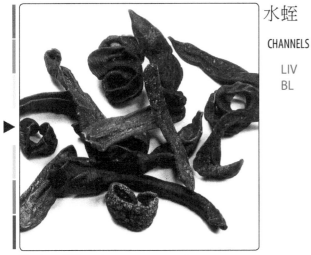

CHANNELS

LIV
BL

Hirudo seu Whitmania
salty, bitter, neutral, slightly toxic

sī guā luò (Dried Skeleton of Vegetable Sponge)

丝瓜络

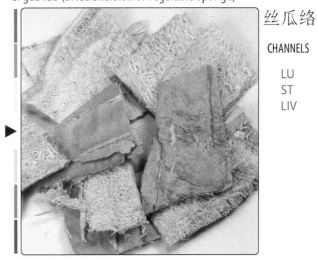

CHANNELS

LU
ST
LIV

Fasciculus Vascularis Luffae
sweet, neutral

sū mù (Sappan Wood)

苏木

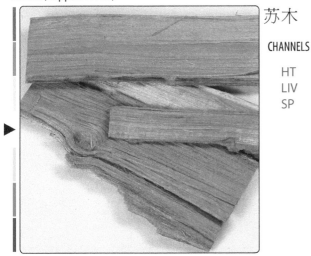

CHANNELS

HT
LIV
SP

Lignum Sappan
sweet, salty, neutral, slightly spicy

táo rén (Peach Kernel)

桃仁

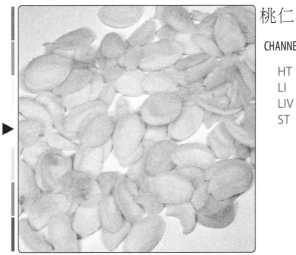

CHANNELS

HT
LI
LIV
ST

Semen Pruni Persicae
bitter, sweet, neutral

Herbs that Invigorate Blood and Remove Stagnation

wǎ lèng zǐ (Cockle Shell, Ark Shell)

瓦楞子

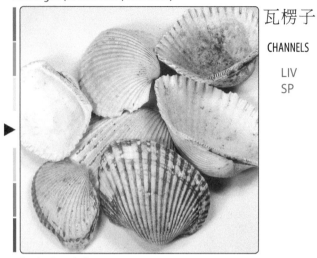

CHANNELS

LIV
SP

Concha Arcae Inflatae
sweet, salty, neutral

wáng bù liú xíng (Vaccaria Seeds)

王不留行

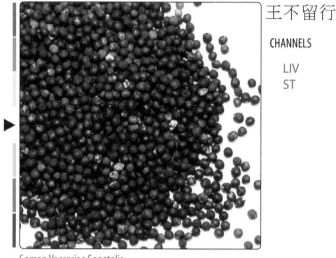

CHANNELS

LIV
ST

Semen Vaccariae Segetalis
bitter, neutral

wǔ líng zhī (Flying Squirrel Feces)

五灵脂

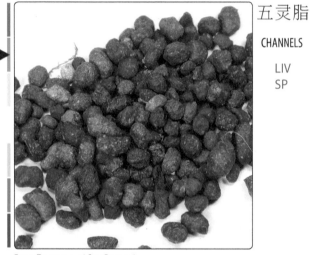

CHANNELS

LIV
SP

Feces Trogopterori Seu Pteromi
bitter, sweet, warm

xuè jié (Dragon's Blood Resin)

血竭

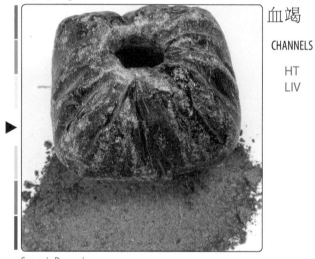

CHANNELS

HT
LIV

Sanguis Draconis
sweet, salty, neutral

yán hú suǒ (Corydalis Rhizome)

延胡索

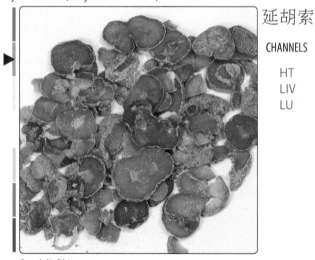

CHANNELS

HT
LIV
LU

Corydalis Rhizome
spicy, bitter, warm

yì mǔ cǎo (Chinese Motherwort)

益母草

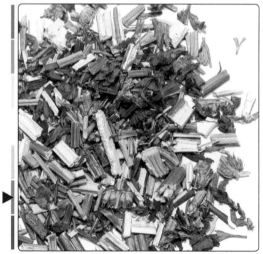

CHANNELS

HT
LIV
BL
PER

Herba Leonuri Heterophylli
spicy, bitter, slightly cold

yù jīn (Tumeric Tuber)

郁金

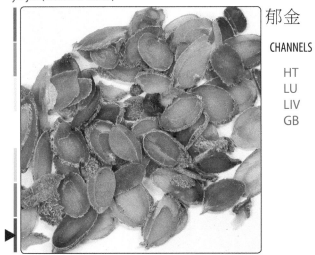

CHANNELS

HT
LU
LIV
GB

Tuber Curcumae
spicy, bitter, cold

zé lán (Bugleweed)

泽兰

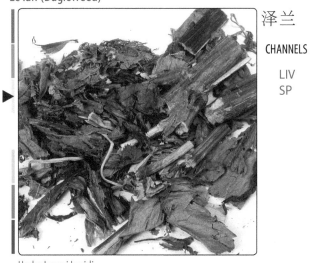

CHANNELS

LIV
SP

Herba Lycopi Lucidi
bitter, spicy, slightly warm, aromatic

bì bá (Long Pepper Fruit)

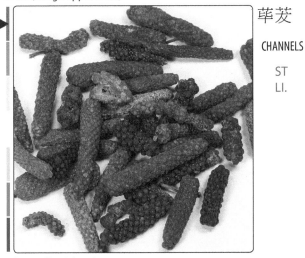

荜茇

CHANNELS

ST
LI.

Fructus Piperis Longi
spicy, hot

chuān jiāo (Fruit of Szechuan Pepper)

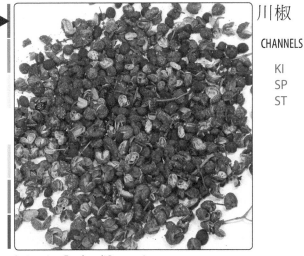

川椒

CHANNELS

KI
SP
ST

Pericarpium Zanthoxyli Bungeani
spicy, hot, slightly toxic

dīng xiāng (Clove Flower Bud)

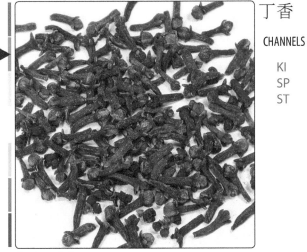

丁香

CHANNELS

KI
SP
ST

Flos Caryophylli
spicy, warm

fù zi (Processed Aconite)

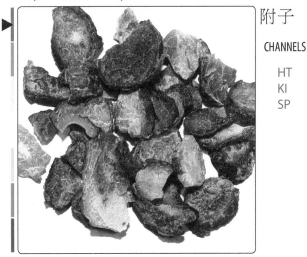

附子

CHANNELS

HT
KI
SP

Radix Lateralis Praeparatus Aconiti Carmichaeli
spicy, hot, toxic

gān jiāng (Dried Ginger Rhizome)

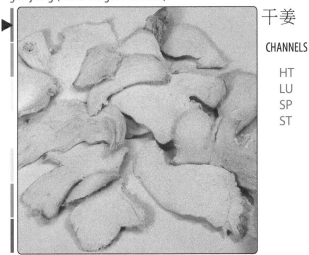

干姜

CHANNELS

HT
LU
SP
ST

dry Rhizoma Zingiberis
spicy, hot

gāo liáng jiāng (Lesser Galangal Rhizome)

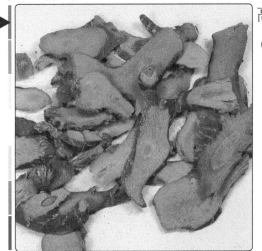

高良姜

CHANNELS

SP
ST

Rhizoma Alpiniae Officinari
spicy, hot

Herbs that Warm the Interior and Expel Cold

hú jiāo (Black Pepper)

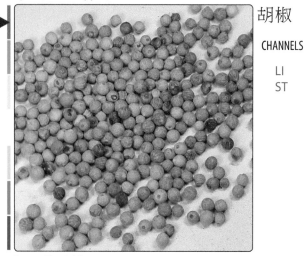

胡椒

CHANNELS

LI
ST

Fructus Piperis Nigri
spicy, hot

ròu guì (Inner Brack or Saigon Cinnamon)

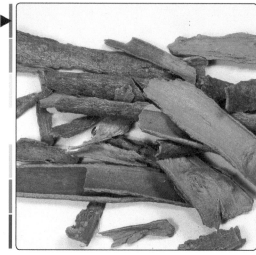

肉桂

CHANNELS

HT
KI
LIV
SP

Cortex Cinnamomi Cassiae
spicy, sweet, hot

wú zhū yú (Evodia Fruit)

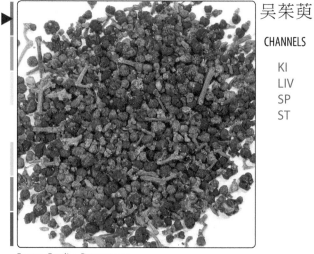

吴茱萸

CHANNELS

KI
LIV
SP
ST

Fructus Evodiae Rutaecarpae
spicy, bitter, hot, slightly toxic, very dry

xiǎo huí xiāng (Fennel Fruit)

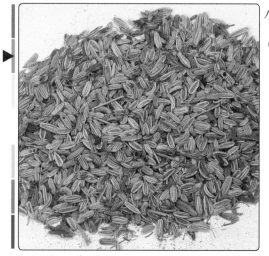

小茴香

CHANNELS

LIV
KI
SP
ST

Fructus Foeniculi Vulgaris
spicy, warm

bái zhú (White Atractylodes Rhizome)

白术

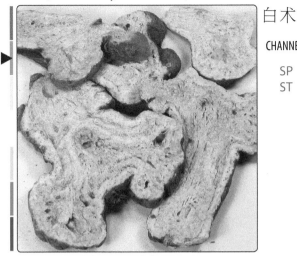

CHANNELS

SP
ST

Rhizoma Atractylodis Macrocephalae
bitter, sweet, warm

dà zǎo (Date, Jujube)

大枣

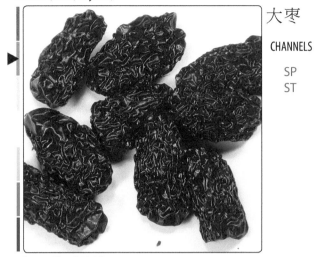

CHANNELS

SP
ST

Fructus Zizyphi Jujubae
sweet, warm

dǎng shēn (Codonopsis Root)

党参

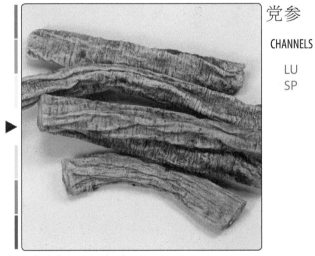

CHANNELS

LU
SP

Radix Codonopsitis Pilosulae
sweet, neutral

fēng mì (Honey)

蜂蜜

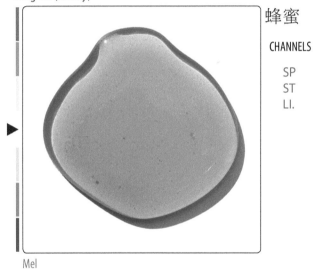

CHANNELS

SP
ST
LI.

Mel
sweet, neutral

gān cǎo (Licorice Root)

甘草

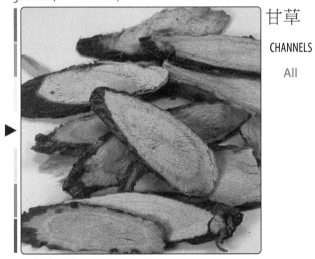

CHANNELS

All

Radix Glycyrrhizae
sweet, neutral

huáng jīng (Siberian Solomon Seal Rhizome, Polygonatum)

黄精

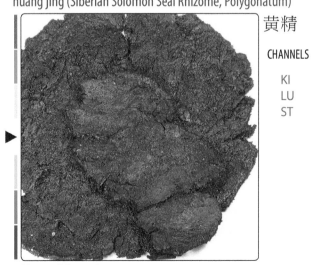

CHANNELS

KI
LU
ST

Rhizoma Polygonati
sweet, neutral

huáng qí (Astragalus)

黄芪

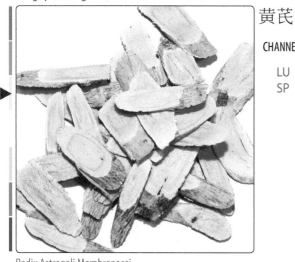

CHANNELS

LU
SP

Radix Astragali Membranacei
sweet, slightly warm

rén shēn (Ginseng Root)

人参

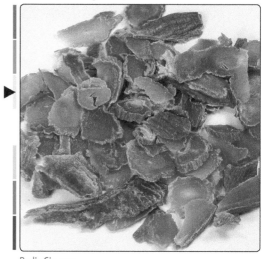

CHANNELS

LU
SP

Radix Ginseng
sweet, slightly bitter, slightly warm

shān yao (Chinese Yam Rhizome, Dioscorea)

山药

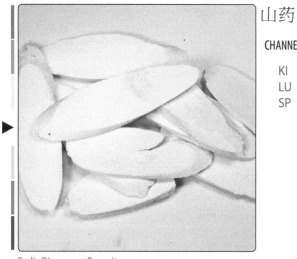

CHANNELS

KI
LU
SP

Radix Dioscoreae Oppositae
sweet, neutral

tài zǐ shēn (Pseudostellaria)

太子参

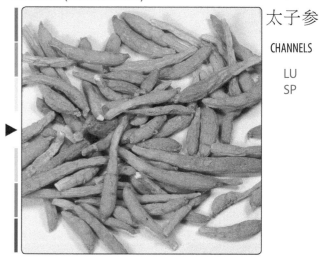

CHANNELS

LU
SP

Radix Pseudostellariae
sweet, slightly bitter, neutral

yí táng (Barley Malt Sugar, Maltose)

饴糖

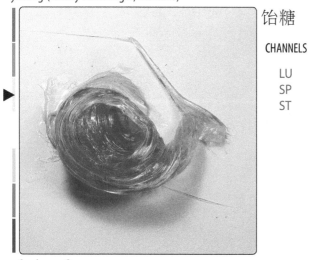

CHANNELS

LU
SP
ST

Saccharum Granorum
sweet, slightly warm

zhì gān cǎo (Honey Fried Licorice Root)

炙甘草

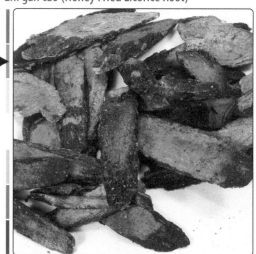

CHANNELS

All

Radix Glycyrrhizae
sweet, warm

bái sháo (White Peony Root)

白芍

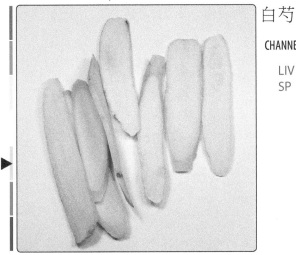

CHANNELS

LIV
SP

Radix Albus Paeoniae Lactiflorae
bitter, sour, cool

dāng guī (Chinese Angelica Root)

当归

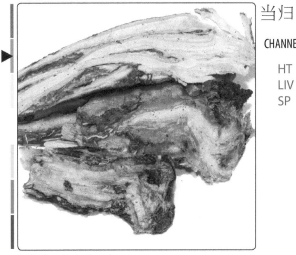

CHANNELS

HT
LIV
SP

Radix Angelicae Sinensis
sweet, spicy, bitter, warm

ē jiāo (Ass Hide Glue, Donkey Hide Gelatin)

阿胶

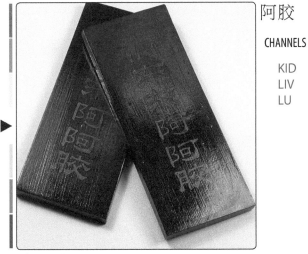

CHANNELS

KID
LIV
LU

Gelatinum Corii Asini
sweet, neutral

gǒu qǐ zǐ (Chinese Wolfberry Fruit, Matrimony Vine Fruit)

枸杞子

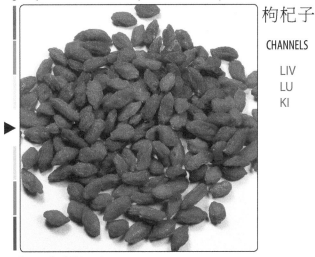

CHANNELS

LIV
LU
KI

Fructus Lycii Chinensis
sweet, neutral

hé shǒu wū (Fleeceflower Root, Ho Shou Wu, Polygonum)

何首乌

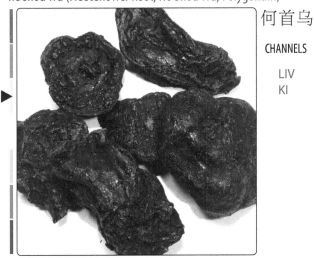

CHANNELS

LIV
KI

Radix Polygoni Multiflori
bitter, sweet, astringent, slightly warm

lóng yǎn ròu (Flesh of the Longan Fruit)

龙眼肉

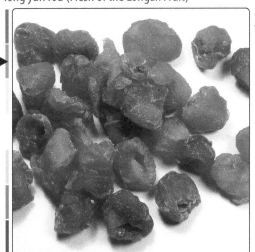

CHANNELS

HT
SP

Arillus Euphoriae Longanae
sweet, warm

sāng shèn (Mulberry Fruit Spike, Morus Fruit)

桑葚

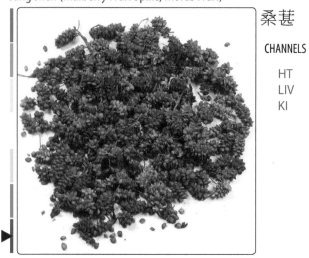

CHANNELS

HT
LIV
KI

Fructus Mori Albae
sweet, cold

shú dì huáng (Chinese Foxglove Root, Steamed with Water or Alcohol)

熟地黃

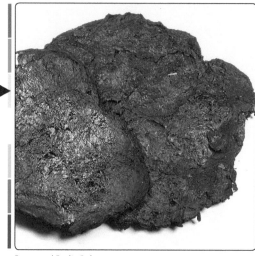

CHANNELS

LIV
KI
(HT)

Processed Radix Rehmanniae
sweet, slightly warm

bā jǐ tiān (Morinda Root)

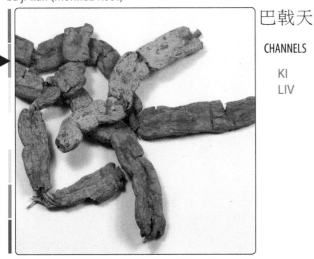

巴戟天

CHANNELS

KI
LIV

Morindae Officinalis Radix
spicy, sweet, warm

bǔ gǔ zhī (Psoralea Fruit)

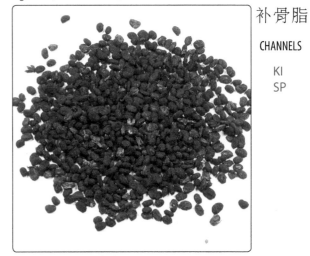

补骨脂

CHANNELS

KI
SP

Fructus Psoraleae Corylifoliae
spicy, bitter, very warm

dōng chóng xià cǎo (Cordyceps, Chinese Caterpillar Fungus)

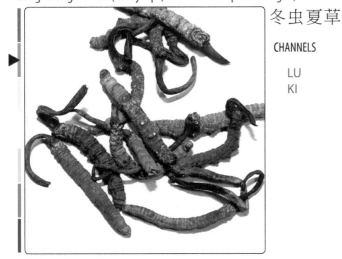

冬虫夏草

CHANNELS

LU
KI

Cordyceps Chinensis
sweet, warm

dù zhòng (Eucommia Bark)

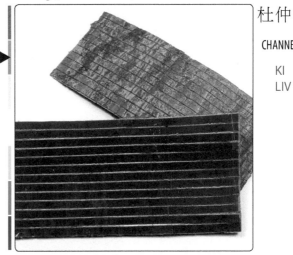

杜仲

CHANNELS

KI
LIV

Cortex Eucommiae Ulmoidis
sweet, slightly spicy, warm

gǒu jǐ (Chain Fern Rhizome)

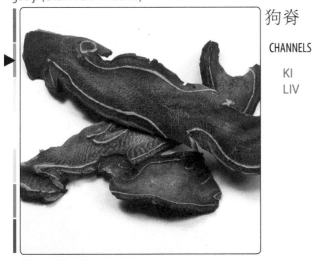

狗脊

CHANNELS

KI
LIV

Rhizoma Cibotii Barometsis
bitter, sweet, warm

gǔ suì bǔ (Drynaria Rhizome)

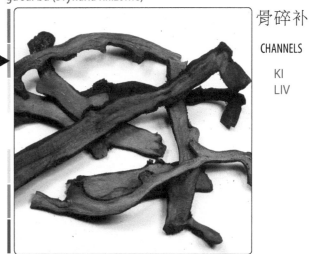

骨碎补

CHANNELS

KI
LIV

Radix Drynariae
bitter, warm

Herbs that Tonify Yang

hǎi mǎ (Sea Horse)

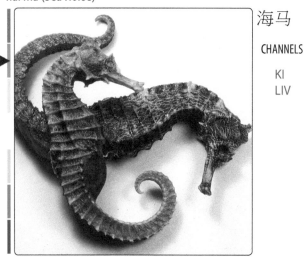

海马

CHANNELS

KI
LIV

Hippocampus
sweet, salty, warm

lù jiǎo jiāo (Deer Horn Gelatin)

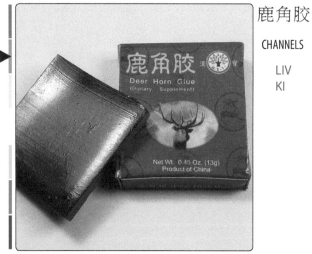

鹿角胶

CHANNELS

LIV
KI

Gelatinum Cornu Cervi
sweet, salty, warm

shā yuàn zǐ (Astragalus Seed, Flattened Milkvetch Seed)

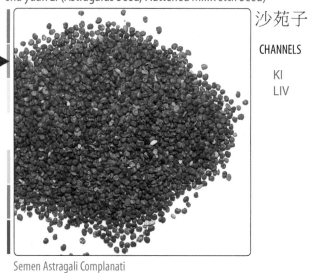

沙苑子

CHANNELS

KI
LIV

Semen Astragali Complanati
sweet, warm

jiǔ cài zi (Chinese Leek/Onion Seed)

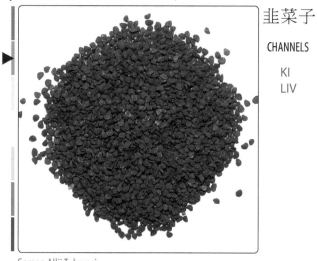

韭菜子

CHANNELS

KI
LIV

Semen Allii Tuberosi
spicy, sweet, warm

ròu cōng róng (Fleshy Stem of the Broomrape)

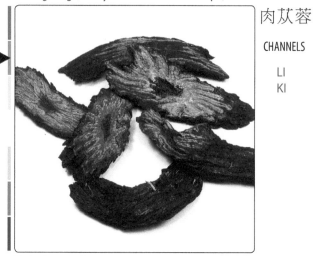

肉苁蓉

CHANNELS

LI
KI

Herba Cistanchis Deserticolae
sweet, salty, warm

suǒ yáng (Fleshy Stem of Cynomorium)

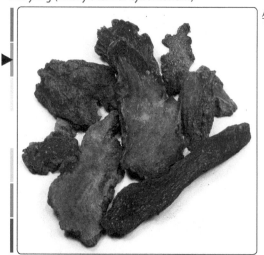

锁阳

CHANNELS

LI
KI
LIV

Herba Cynomorii Songarici
sweet, warm

tù sī zǐ (Chinese Dodder Seeds)

菟丝子

CHANNELS

KI
LIV

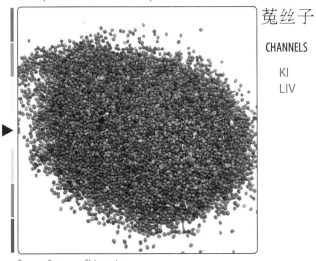

Semen Cuscutae Chinensis
spicy, sweet, neutral

xiān máo (Golden Eye Grass Rhizome)

仙茅

CHANNELS

KI
LIV

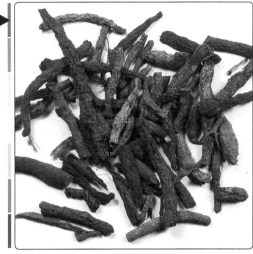

Rhizoma Curculiginis Orchioidis
spicy, hot, toxic

xù duàn (Japanese Teasel Root)

续断

CHANNELS

KI
LIV

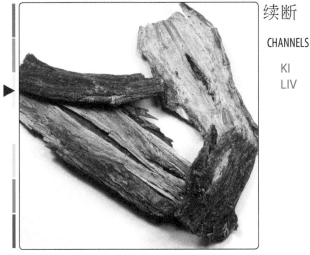

Radix Dipsaci
bitter, spicy, slightly warm

yì zhī rén (Black Cardamom, Alpinia Oxyphylla Fruit)

益知仁

CHANNELS

KI
SP

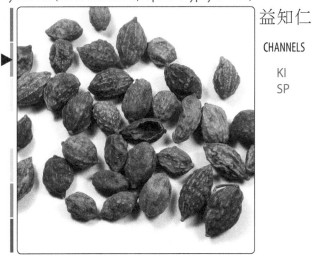

Fructus Alpiniae Oxyphyllae
spicy, warm

yīn yáng huò (Aerial Parts of Epimedium)

阴阳霍

CHANNELS

KI
LIV

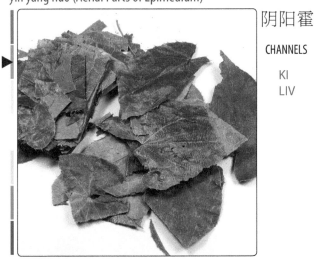

Herba Epimedii
spicy, sweet, warm

zǐ hé chē (Human Placenta)

紫河车

CHANNELS

LIV
LU
KI

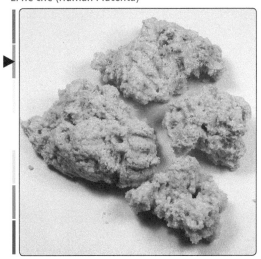

Placenta Hominis
sweet, salty, warm

băi hé (Lily Bulb)

百合

CHANNELS

HT
LU

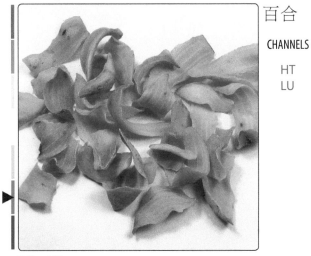

Bulbus Lilii
sweet, slightly bitter, slightly cold

biē jiă (Chinese Soft Shelled Turtle Shell)

鳖甲

CHANNELS

LIV
SP

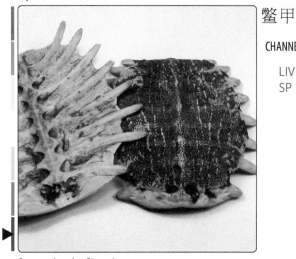

Carapax Amydae Sinensis
salty, cold

guī băn (Fresh Water Turtle Shell, Testudinis)

龟板

CHANNELS

HT
KI
LIV

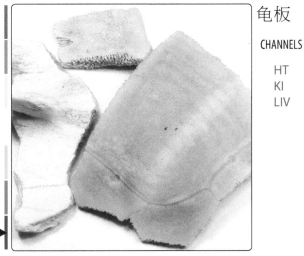

Plastrum Testudinis
salty, sweet, cold

hàn lián căo (Eclipta)

旱莲草

CHANNELS

KI
LIV

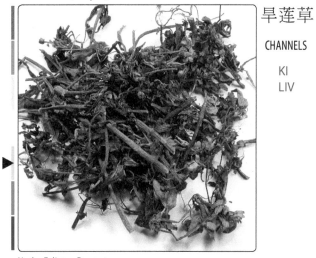

Herba Ecliptae Prostratae
sweet, sour, cool

hēi zhī ma (Black Sesame Seeds)

黑芝麻

CHANNELS

KI
LIV

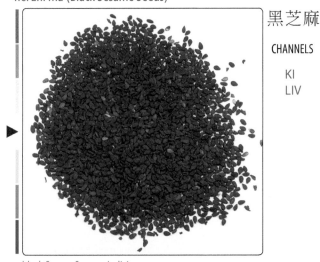

black Semen Sesame Indici
sweet, neutral

luó hàn guŏ (Momordica Fruit)

罗汉果

CHANNELS

LU
LI
(SP)

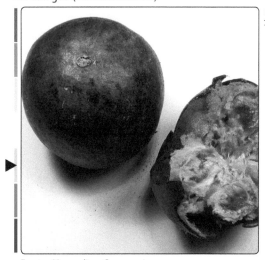

Fructus Momordicae Grosvenori
sweet, cool (or neutral)

mài mén dōng (Ophiopogon Tuber)

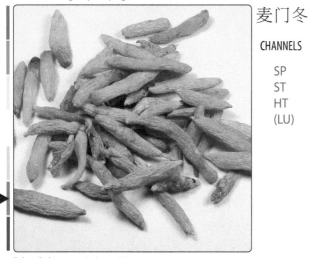

麦门冬

CHANNELS

SP
ST
HT
(LU)

Tuber Ophiopogonis Japonici
sweet, slightly bitter, slightly cold

nu zhēn zǐ (Privet Fruit, Ligustrum)

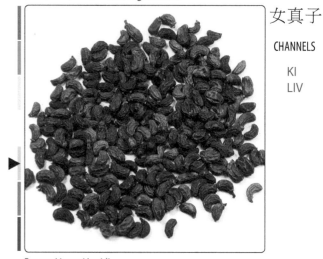

女真子

CHANNELS

KI
LIV

Fructus Ligustri Lucidi
bitter, sweet, cool (or neutral)

sāng jì shēng (Mulberry Mistletoe Stems)

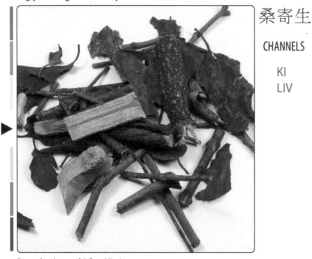

桑寄生

CHANNELS

KI
LIV

Ramulus Loranthi Seu Visci
bitter, neutral

shí hú (Dendrobium Stem)

you gua shi hu shown

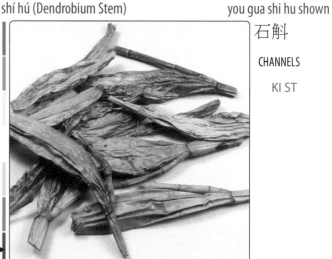

石斛

CHANNELS

KI ST

Herba Dendrobii
sweet, slightly salty, bland, cold

tiān mén dōng (Asparagus Tuber)

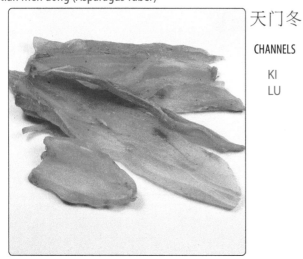

天门冬

CHANNELS

KI
LU

Tuber Asparagi Cochinensis
sweet, bitter, very cold

xī yáng shēn (American Ginseng Root)

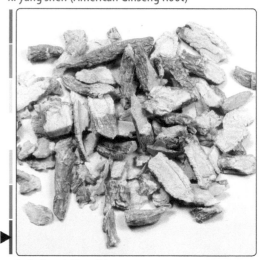

西洋参

CHANNELS

HT
KI
LU

Radix Panacis Qinquifolii
sweet, slightly bitter, cold

yín ěr (Fruiting Body of Tremella, Wood Ear)

银耳

CHANNELS

LU
ST

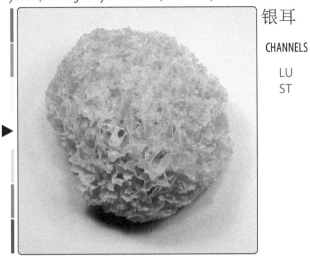

Fructificatio Tremellae Fuciformis
sweet, bland, neutral

yù zhú (Solomon's Seal Rhizome, Polygonatum)

玉竹

CHANNELS

LU
ST

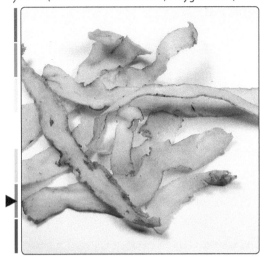

Rhizoma Polygonati Odorati
sweet, slightly cold

bái guǒ (Ginkgo Nut)

白果

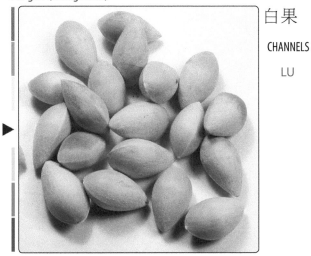

CHANNELS

LU

Semen Ginkgonis Bilobae
sweet, bitter, astringent, neutral, slightly toxic

chūn pí (Ailanthus Bark or Root Bark)

椿皮

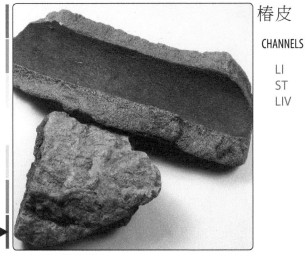

CHANNELS

LI
ST
LIV

Cortex Ailanthi Altissimae
bitter, astringent, cold

fú xiǎo mài (Wheat Grain (Not Yet Ripe))

浮小麦

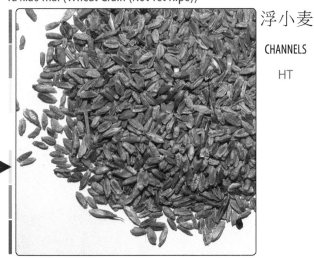

CHANNELS

HT

Fructus Levis Tritici Aestivi
sweet, salty, cool

chì shí zhī (Halloysite, Kaolin)

赤石脂

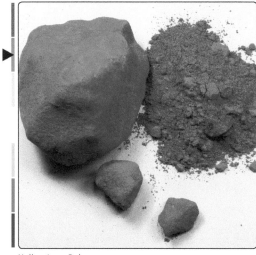

CHANNELS

ST
LI.
(SP)

Hallyositum Rubrum
sweet, sour, astringent, warm

fù pén zǐ (Chinese Rasberry)

覆盆子

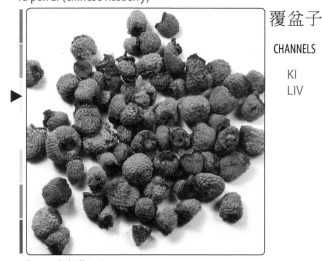

CHANNELS

KI
LIV

Fructus Rubi Chingii
sweet, astringent, slightly warm

hǎi piāo xiāo (Cuttlefish Bone, Cuttlebone)

海螵蛸

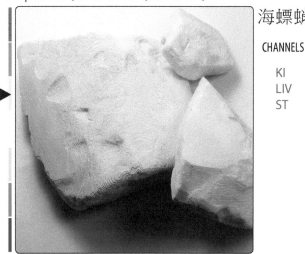

CHANNELS

KI
LIV
ST

Os Sepiae Seu Sepiellae
salty, astringent, slightly warm

Herbs that Astringe, Stabilize, Bind

hè zǐ (Myrobalan Fruit)

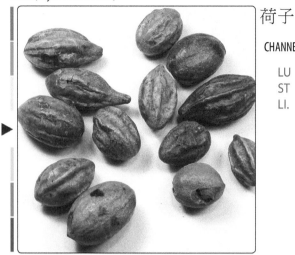

荷子

CHANNELS

LU
ST
LI.

Fructus Terminaliae Chebulae
bitter, sour, astringent, neutral

jīn yīng zǐ (Cherokee Rosehip)

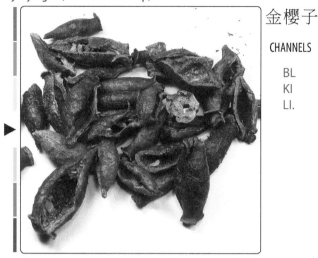

金樱子

CHANNELS

BL
KI
LI.

Fructus Rosae Laevigatae
sour, astringent, neutral

lián xū (Lotus Stamen)

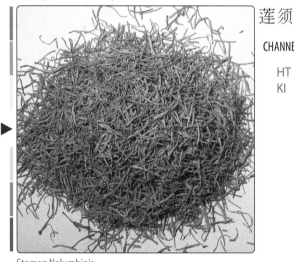

莲须

CHANNELS

HT
KI

Stamen Nelumbinis
sweet, astringent, neutral

lián zǐ (Lotus Seed)

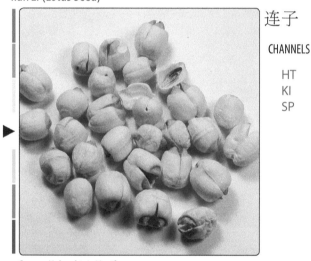

连子

CHANNELS

HT
KI
SP

Semen Nelumbinis Nuciferae
sweet, astringent, neutral

má huáng gēn (Ephedra Root)

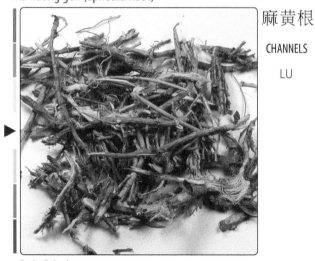

麻黄根

CHANNELS

LU

Radix Ephedrae
sweet, neutral

nuò dào gēn xū (Glutinous Rice Root)

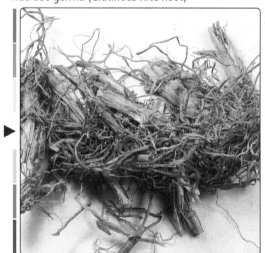

糯稻根鬚

CHANNELS

KI
LIV
LU

Radix Oryzae Glutinosae
sweet, neutral

qiàn shí (Euryale Seeds)

芡实

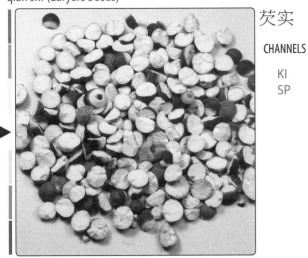

CHANNELS

KI
SP

Semen Euryalis Ferocis
sweet, astringent, neutral

ròu dòu kòu (Nutmeg Seeds)

肉豆蔻

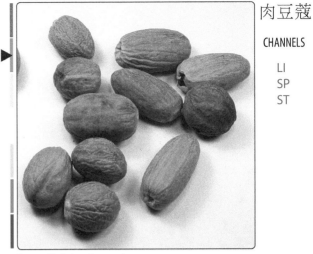

CHANNELS

LI
SP
ST

Semen Myristicae Fragrantis
spicy, warm

sāng piāo xiāo (Mantis Egg Case)

桑螵蛸

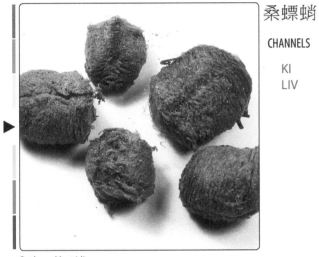

CHANNELS

KI
LIV

Ootheca Mantidis
sweet, salty, neutral

shān zhū yú (Asiatic Cornelian Cherry Fruit, Cornus)

山茱萸

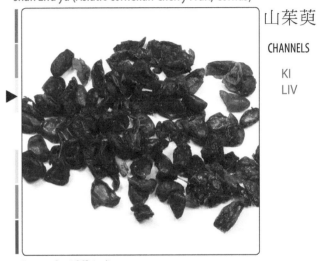

CHANNELS

KI
LIV

Fructus Corni Officinalis
sour, slightly warm

wǔ bèi zǐ (Gallnet of Chinese Sumac)

五倍子

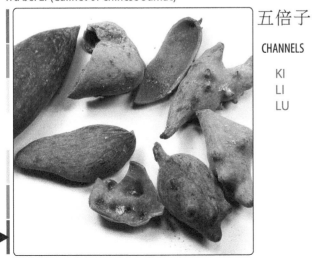

CHANNELS

KI
LI
LU

Galla Rhois
sour, salty, cold

wū méi (Mume Fruit)

乌梅

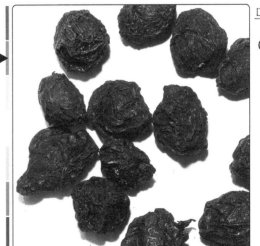

CHANNELS

LI
LIV
LU
SP

Fructus Pruni Mume
sour, warm

wǔ wèi zǐ (Schisandra Fruit) nan wu wei zi shown

五味子

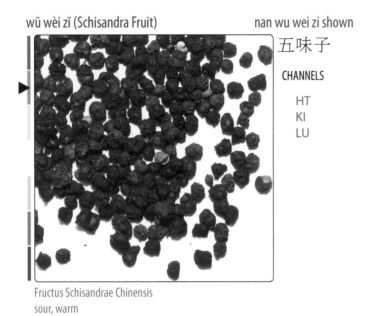

CHANNELS

HT
KI
LU

Fructus Schisandrae Chinensis
sour, warm

cí shí (Magnetite)

磁石

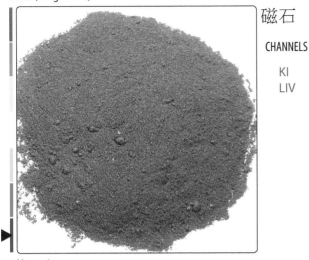

CHANNELS

KI
LIV

Magnetitum
spicy, salty, cold

dài zhě shí (Hematite)

代赭石

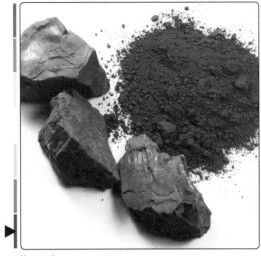

CHANNELS

HT
LIV
PER

Haematitum
bitter, cold

hǔ pò (Amber)

琥魄

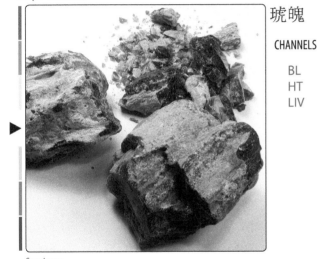

CHANNELS

BL
HT
LIV

Succinum
sweet, neutral

lóng chǐ (Fossilized Mammal Teeth)

龙齿

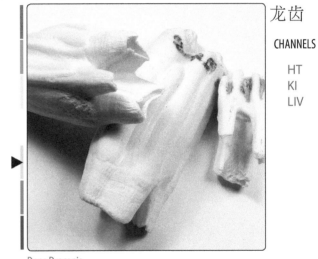

CHANNELS

HT
KI
LIV

Dens Draconis
astringent, cool

lóng gǔ (Fossilized Mammal Bones)

龙骨

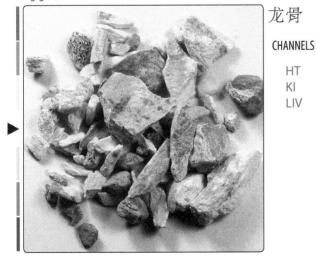

CHANNELS

HT
KI
LIV

Os Draconis
sweet, astringent, neutral

mǔ lì (Oyster Shell)

牡蛎

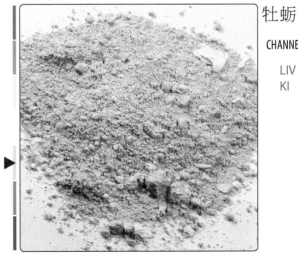

CHANNELS

LIV
KI

Concha Ostreae
salty, astringent, cool

Visual Materia Medica of Chinese Herbs, Sacred Lotus Arts

Substances that Anchor, Settle, and Calm the Spirit

zhēn zhū mǔ (Mother of Pearl)

珍珠母

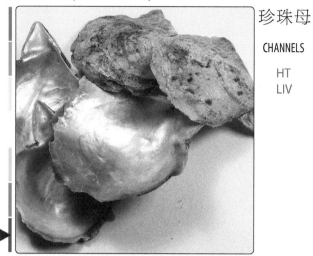

CHANNELS

HT
LIV

Concha Margaratiferae
sweet, salty, cold

zǐ shí yīng (Flourite)

紫石英

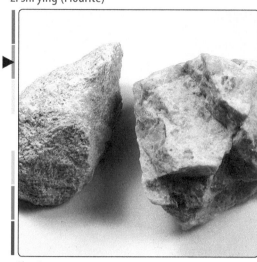

CHANNELS

HT
LIV

Fluoritum
sweet, warm

bǎi zǐ rén (Arbor Vitae Seed, Biota Seed)

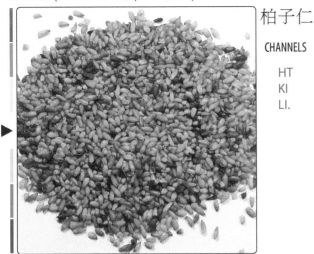

柏子仁

CHANNELS

HT
KI
LI.

Semen Platycladi
sweet, neutral

hé huàn huā (Mimosa Tree Flower)

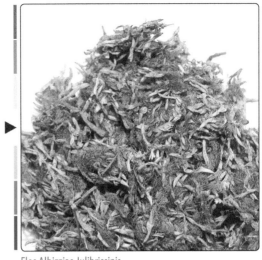

合换花

CHANNELS

HT
LIV

Flos Albizziae Julibrissinis
sweet, neutral

hé huān pí (Mimosa Tree Bark)

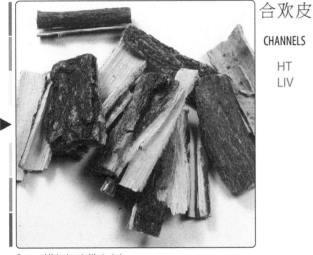

合欢皮

CHANNELS

HT
LIV

Cortex Albizziae Julibrissinis
sweet, neutral

suān zǎo rén (Sour Jujube Seed, Zizyphus - Raw Herb Shown)

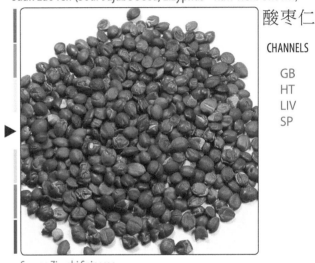

酸枣仁

CHANNELS

GB
HT
LIV
SP

Semen Zizyphi Spinosae
sweet, sour, neutral

yè jiāo téng (Fleeceflower Vine, Polygonum Vine)

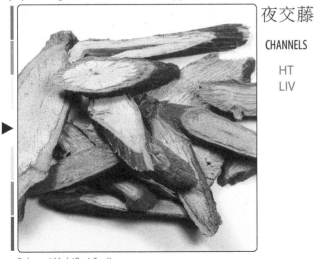

夜交藤

CHANNELS

HT
LIV

Polygoni Multiflori Caulis
sweet, slightly bitter, neutral

yuán zhì (Chinese Senega Root)

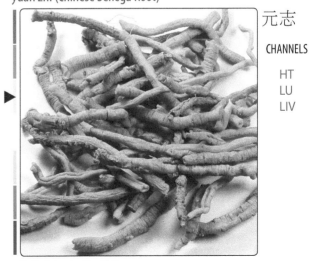

元志

CHANNELS

HT
LU
LIV

Radix Polygalae Tenuifoliae
bitter, spicy, slightly warm

bīng piàn (Borneol)

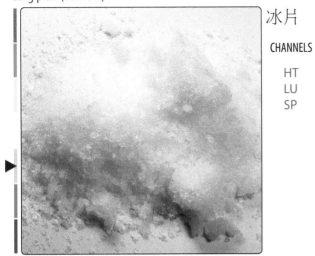

冰片

CHANNELS

HT
LU
SP

Borneolum
spicy, bitter, cool

shí chāng pú (Sweetflag Rhizome)

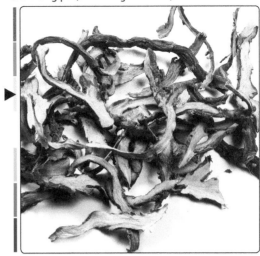

石菖蒲

CHANNELS

HT
ST

Rhizoma Acori Graminei
spicy, slightly warm, aromatic

bái jí lí (Caltrop Fruit, Tribulus)

白蒺藜

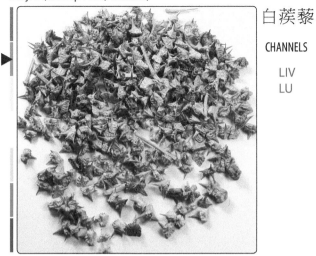

CHANNELS

LIV
LU

Fructus Tribuli Terrestris
spicy, bitter, warm

dì lóng (Earthworm)

地龙

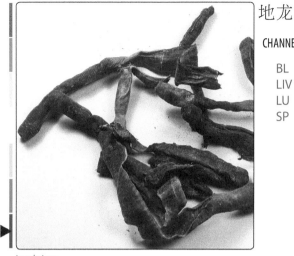

CHANNELS

BL
LIV
LU
SP

Lumbricus
salty, cold

gōu téng (Gambir Vine Stems and Thorns)

钩藤

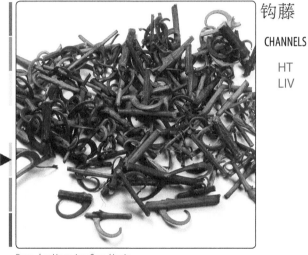

CHANNELS

HT
LIV

Ramulus Uncariae Cum Uncis
sweet, cool

jiāng cán (Body of Sick Silkworm)

僵蚕

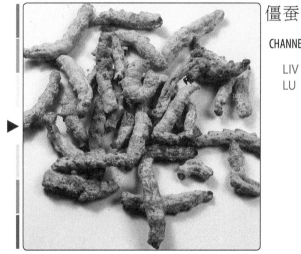

CHANNELS

LIV
LU

Bombyx Batryticatus
spicy, salty, neutral

líng yáng jiǎo (Antelope Horn)

羚羊角

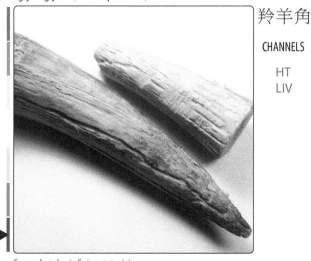

CHANNELS

HT
LIV

Comu Antelopis Saiga-tatarici
salty, cold

quán xiē (Scorpion, Buthus)

全蝎

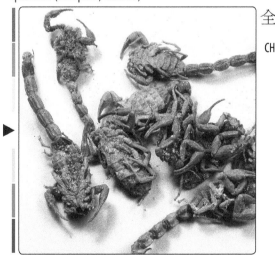

CHANNELS

LIV

Buthus Martensis
salty, spicy, neutral, toxic

shí jué míng (Abalone Shell)

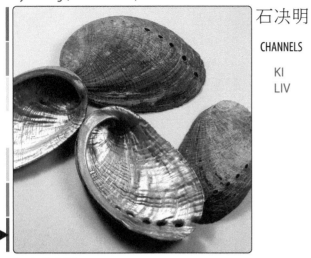

石决明

CHANNELS

KI
LIV

Concha Haliotidis
salty, cold

tiān má (Gastrodia Rhizome)

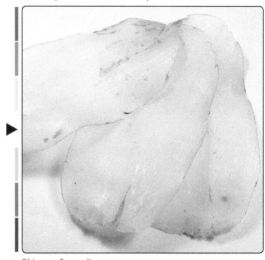

天麻

CHANNELS

LIV

Rhizoma Gastrodiae
sweet, neutral

wú gōng (Centipede)

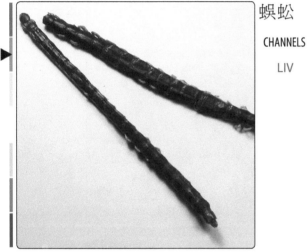

蜈蚣

CHANNELS

LIV

Scolopendra Subspinipes
spicy, warm, toxic

bīng láng (Betel Nut)

槟榔

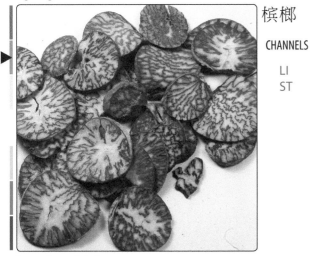

CHANNELS

LI
ST

Semen Arecae Catechu
spicy, bitter, warm

cháng shān (Dichroa Root)

常山

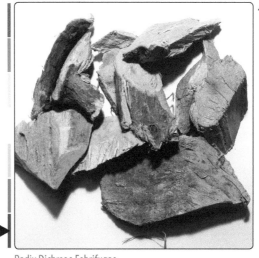

CHANNELS

HT
LIV
LU

Radix Dichroae Febrifugae
bitter, spicy, cold, toxic

fěi zi (Torreya Seeds)

榧子

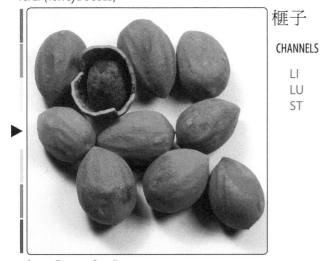

CHANNELS

LI
LU
ST

Semen Torreyae Grandis
sweet, astringent, neutral

guàn zhòng (Dryopteris Root)

贯众

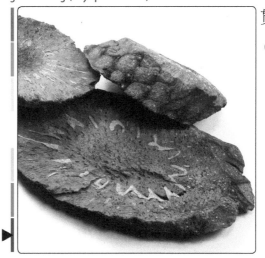

CHANNELS

LIV
SP

Rhizoma Guanchong
bitter, cold

hè shī (Carpesium Fruit)

鹤虱

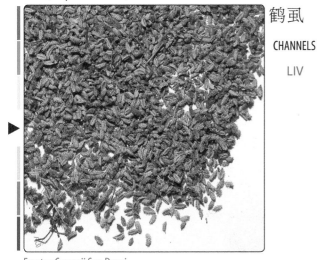

CHANNELS

LIV

Fructus Carpesii Seu Dauci
bitter, spicy, neutral, slightly toxic

léi wán (Fruiting Body of Omphalia)

雷丸

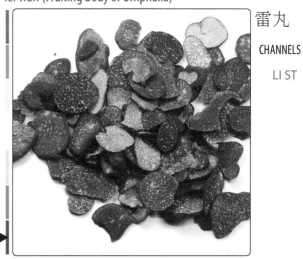

CHANNELS

LI ST

Scierotium Omphaliae Lapidescentis
bitter, cold, slightly toxic

shǐ jūn zǐ (Rangoon Creeper Fruit with Seeds)

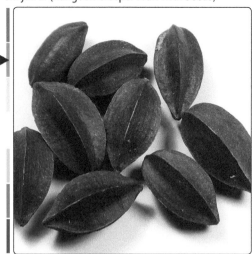

使君子

CHANNELS

SP
ST

Fructus Quisqualis
sweet, warm

ér chá (Paste from Dried Conc. Decoction of Black or Brown Cutch)

儿茶

CHANNELS

LU

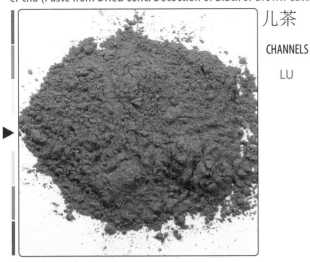

Pasta Acaciae Seu Uncariae
bitter, astringent, neutral

mǎ qián zǐ (Nux Vomica Seeds)

马钱子

CHANNELS

LIV
SP

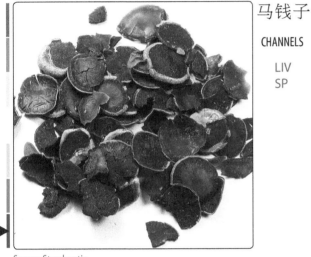

Semen Strychnotis
bitter, cold, toxic

péng shā (Borax)

硼砂

CHANNELS

LU
ST

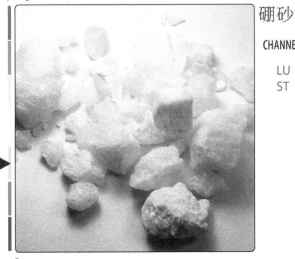

Borax
sweet, salty, cool

liú huáng (Sulpher)

硫磺

CHANNELS

KI LI
PER

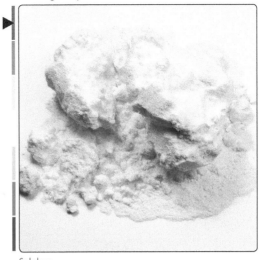

Sulphur
sour, hot, toxic

míng fán (Alum)

明矾

CHANNELS

LI
LIV
LU
SP
ST

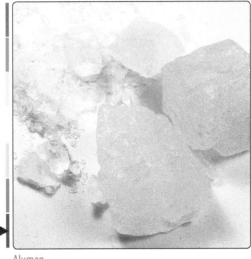

Alumen
sour, astringent, cold

shān cí gū (Bulb of Chinese Tulip)

山茨菇

CHANNELS

LIV
ST

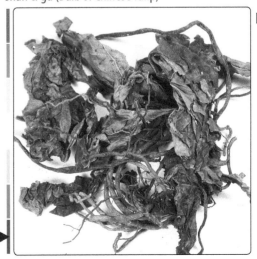

Pseudobulbus Shancigu
sweet, cold, slightly toxic

Substances for External Application

shé chuáng zǐ (Cnidium Seeds)

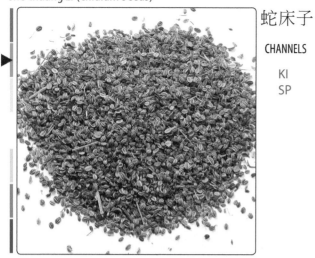

蛇床子

CHANNELS

KI
SP

Fructus Cnidii Monnieni
spicy, bitter, warm

xióng huáng (Realgar)

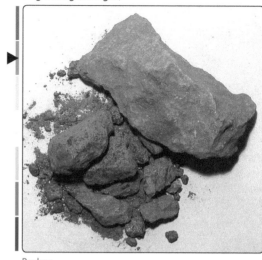

雄黄

CHANNELS

HT
LIV
ST

Realgar
spicy, bitter, warm, toxic

zhāng nǎo (Camphor)

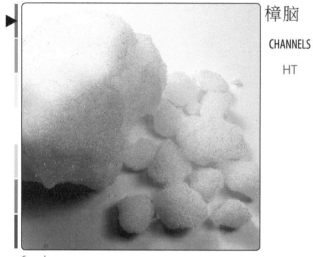

樟腦

CHANNELS

HT

Camphora
spicy, hot, toxic

Pinyin Name Index

tíng lì zǐ	15	yù jīn	20
tōng cǎo	11	yù lǐ rén	09
tǔ fú líng	06	yù mǐ xū	11
niú xī	06	yú xīng cǎo	06
tù sī zǐ	24	yù zhú	25
wǎ lèng zǐ	20	yuán hu	10
wáng bù liú xíng	20	yuán zhì	28
wēi líng xiān	12	zào jiǎo cì	14
wǔ bèi zǐ	26	zé lán	20
wú gōng	30	zé xiè	11
wǔ jiā pí	12	zhāng nǎo	32
wǔ líng zhī	20	Zhè bèi mǔ	13
wū méi	26	zhēn zhū mǔ	27
wǔ wèi zǐ	26	zhì gān cǎo	22
wū yào	18	zhǐ ké	18
wú zhū yú	21	zhī mǔ	03
xī jiǎo	04	zhǐ shí	18
xī xiān cǎo	12	zhì tiān nán xīng	14
xì xīn	01	zhī zi	03
xī yáng shēn	25	zhū líng	11
xià kū cǎo	03	zhú rù	13
xiān hè cǎo	19	zǐ cǎo	04
xiān máo	24	zǐ hé chē	24
xiāng fù	18	zǐ huā dì dīng	06
xiāng rú	01	zǐ shí yīng	27
xiǎo huí xiāng	21	zǐ sū gěng	01
xiè bái	18	zǐ sū yè	01
xīn yí	01	zǐ sū zǐ	15
xìng rén	15	zǐ wǎn	15
xióng huáng	32		
xù duàn	24		
xuàn fù huā	14		
xuán shēn	04		
xuè jié	20		
xiě yú tàn	19		
yā dàn zǐ	06		
yán hú suǒ	20		
yè jiāo téng	28		
yě jú huā	06		
yè míng shā	03		
yì mǔ cǎo	20		
yí táng	22		
yì yǐ rén	11		
yì zhī rén	24		
yīn chái hú	04		
yīn chén	11		
yín ěr	25		
yīn yáng huò	24		

Common English Name Index

Latin Name Index

Latin Name Index

CPSIA information can be obtained
at www.ICGtesting.com
Printed in the USA
LVHW070025291220
675296LV00003B/37